Get Through
MRCPCH Part 1: BOFs and EMQs

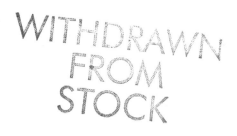

To my son Abdul Hakim

Get Through
MRCPCH Part I: BOFs and EMQs

Nagi Giumma Barakat MB, BCh, MRCPCH, MSc Epilepsy, CCST, FRCPCH

Consultant Paediatrician, Hillingdon Hospital, London, UK
Honorary Consultant, Neurology Department,
Great Ormond Street Hospital for Sick Children,
London, UK

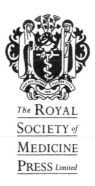

The ROYAL
SOCIETY *of*
MEDICINE
PRESS *Limited*

Published by the Royal Society of Medicine Press Ltd
1 Wimpole Street, London W1G 0AE, UK
Tel: +44 (0)20 7290 2921
Fax: +44 (0)20 7290 2929
Email: publishing@rsm.ac.uk
Website: www.rsmpress.co.uk

British Library Cataloguing in Publication Data
A catalogue record for this book is available from the British Library

ISBN 1-85315-658-2

Distribution in Europe and Rest of World:

Marston Book Services Ltd
PO Box 269
Abingdon
Oxon OX14 4YN, UK
Tel: +44 (0)1235 465500
Fax: +44 (0)1235 465555
Email: direct.order@marston.co.uk

Distribution in the USA and Canada:

Royal Society of Medicine Press Ltd
c/o BookMasters Inc
30 Amberwood Parkway
Ashland, OH 44805, USA
Tel: +1 800 247 6553/+1 800 266 5564
Fax: +1 419 281 6883
Email: orders@bookmasters.com

Distribution in Australia and New Zealand:

Elsevier Australia
30–52 Smidmore Street
Marrikville NSW 2204, Australia
Tel: +61 2 9349 5811
Fax: +61 2 9349 5911
Email: service@elsevier.com.au

Typeset by SR Nova Pvt Ltd, Bangalore, India
Printed and bound in Great Britain by Bell & Bain Ltd, Glasgow

Contents

Preface

This book has been written in response to changes in the MRCPCH entry criteria. It is aimed at both paediatricians in training and those preparing for postgraduate examinations. There are 500 questions, all of which are either Best of Fives (BOFs) or Extended Matching Questions (EMQs), selected according to the revised entry criteria. The questions, and the accompanying notes on conditions, have been written drawing on many resources, as well as on the wide personal experience of the author as a clinican and teacher. The content is intended to be comprehensive and easy to read, with both basic and clinical knowledge applied as much as possible.

My advice to readers is to look at the questions, try to answer them, and then turn to the answers. If you think that you disagree with an answer, go to one of the references and read more about the relevant topic. You may find it helpful to read this book together with colleagues – exchanging views as well as knowledge will help in understanding the questions and solving the problems.

Nagi G Barakat
London

Acknowledgements

I should like to take this opportunity to thank the RSM Press team who helped with this book and their patience for my delay in delivering it on time. Thanks are also due to my secretary Ms Amanda Tisdal and to the junior doctors who reviewed and corrected my mistakes. I am grateful as well to all the other colleagues and family who have given me advice about this subject.

References and further reading

Aicardi J. *Diseases of the Nervous System in Childhood*, 2nd edn. London: MacKeith, 1998.

Behrman RE, Kleigman RM, Nelson WE, Vaughan VC. *Nelson's Textbook of Paediatrics*, 17th edn. London: WB Saunders, 2003.

Bentley R, Lifschitiz C, Lawson M. *Pediatric Gastroentrology and Clinical Nutrition*. Remedica, 2002.

Brook C, Hindmarsh P. *Clinical Pediatric Endocrinology*. Blackwell Sciences (UK), 2001.

Campbell AGM, McIntosh N. *Forfar and Arneil Textbook of Paediatrics*, 6th edn. Edinburgh: Churchill Livingstone, 2002.

Jordan SC, Scott O. *Heart Diseases in Paediatrics*, 3rd edn. Butterworth Heinemann, 1998.

Postlethwaite RJ. *Clinical Paediatric Nephrology*. Bristol: IOPP, 1986.

Accident and Emergency

BOFs

1. **The following are true regarding paediatric A&E except:**

   A The leading reason for A&E Department attendance in young children is infection.

   B Injuries are the second leading cause of morbidity and mortality in children.

   C Most accidents occur within the home setting.

   D In children presenting with seizures, the seizures are mainly secondary to febrile illness.

   E The disintegration of the nuclear family is one factor increasing the demand on medical time.

2. **The following statements are true except:**

   A The function of pre-hospital care is to transfer ill or injured patients to A&E and tertiary-level care services.

   B The availability, free of charge, of a universal national access code (999) is the most effective component in pre-hospital care.

   C In units that combine paediatric and adult patients, paediatric illness recognition and treatment skills may be deficient compared with dedicated paediatric units.

   D In dedicated paediatric units, experience of dealing with major injury and illness is superior to that of units combining in paediatric and adult patients.

   E The nursing staff only, and not the medical staff, should perform triage.

3. **Regarding airway management during resuscitation, the following are true except:**

   A The first step in basic life support for a child found lying on the floor and not moving is airway maintenance.

   B A maintainable airway is defined as one that can be kept open with simple measures, such as the use of an oropharyngeal airway.

   C An unmaintainable airway is one that is still at risk of complete obstruction and necessitates either intubation or the creation of a surgical airway.

   D Any attempt to intubate taking longer than 30 seconds should be abandoned and the child oxygenated with a bag–valve–mask device, pending a second attempt.

   E All sick or injured children require high-flow oxygen.

4. **All of the following are true regarding the management of breathing during resuscitation except:**

   A The efficacy of breathing can be assessed at any time during resuscitation.

   B Respiratory compromise can be characterized by either an increasing or a decreasing work of breathing.

   C If breathing is absent, the child should be intubated immediately.

   D Absent breath sounds and hyper-resonance to percussion on one side suggest the diagnosis of a pneumothorax, which should be confirmed by an urgent portable chest X-ray.

   E Tension pneumothorax should be treated immediately by insertion of a chest drain.

5. **The following statements about the management of circulation during resuscitation are false except:**

   A In a child, the brachial pulse should be palpated in the upper arm.

   B If no pulse is palpable in a child, cardiac massage should be started at a rate of 80–100 bpm.

   C All children with circulatory embarrassment should have an intra-osseous needle inserted immediately into the tibia or femur.

   D Colloids, normal saline and 10% dextrose solutions are equally good in the initial management of circulatory compromise in children.

   E Blood pressure is a reliable sign of circulatory compromise in children.

6. **Regarding cardiac arrest, the following are true except:**

   A Pulseless electrical activity (PEA) is not the commonest form of cardiac arrest in children.

   B Electromechanical dissociation (EMD), and ventricular fibrillation (VF) are three different forms of cardiac arrest in children.

   C The outcome of cardiac arrest in children is worse compared with adults.

   D If cardiac function is restored, children usually recover with no or minimal neurological deficit.

   E Absence of cardiac complexes on the cardiac monitor confirms that the child is in asystole.

7. **In children with cardiac arrest, prolonged resuscitation is indicated in the following clinical situations except:**

   A Poisoning

   B Drowning

   C Unknown cause

   D Hypothermia

   E Post-traumatic cardiac arrest

8. The following drugs may be used or considered in the management of an arrested child with ventricular fibrillation except:

    A Adrenaline
    B Atropine
    C Bretylium
    D Lidocaine (Lignocaine)
    E Bicarbonate

9. One of the following is not a recognized cause of cardiac arrest with pulseless electrical activity:

    A Electrolyte disturbances
    B Hypothermia
    C Cardiac tamponade
    D Tension pneumothorax
    E None of the above

10. The following statements are true regarding the management of major trauma in children except:

    A Spinal cord injury without radiological abnormality (SCIWORA) is not uncommon.
    B In SCIWORA, there is no evidence of fracture, but evidence of subluxation may be present on X-ray.
    C Even if the child is awake and is able to move all four limbs, SCIWORA is still a significant possibility.
    D Sandbags and taping the head to a spinal board are not practically useful to immobilize the head of an unconscious child.
    E The airway should be assessed and opened without moving the cervical spine.

11. In the assessment of a seriously injured child, which one of the following is true?

    A The relatively large head compared with the rest of the body makes the child less vulnerable to head injury than the adult.
    B Pupillary reflexes documented early may alter management significantly.
    C The first assessment does not need to include calculating the Glasgow Coma Scale.
    D Use of a plain X-ray, ultrasound and computed tomography (CT) may help during the primary survey.
    E Bleeding from the ear and nose should be discovered during the primary survey.

12. The following are false regarding the management of poisoned children in the A&E department except:

A Poisoning in children is most common between the second and third years of life.

B The method of choice for children who require gastric decontamination is gastric lavage.

C Administration of syrup of ipecacuanha has been shown to be very effective even several hours after ingestion of the poison.

D Specific antidotes are available for a large number of poisons.

E Most children will not drink charcoal, as it is unpleasant.

13. The following statements are false in acutely ill children except:

A Serious bacterial diseases are common in children aged 3 years and over.

B Meningococcaemia has more or less been eradicated with effective vaccination in the Western world.

C Intussusception is a common surgical emergency in children in the first 3 months of life.

D Epiglottitis has more or less been eradicated with effective vaccination in the Western world.

E Meningitis is one of the common infections in children aged 3 years and over.

14. The only one of the following statements related to very acute sick children is:

A Chest X-ray, urine culture and lumbar puncture must be performed before intravenous antibiotics are administered.

B Most seizure disorders presenting with status epilepticus are due to metabolic defects such as hypoglycaemia or an electrolyte disorder.

C Comatose children can usually maintain their airways.

D Supraventricular tachycardia (SVT) in children usually presents with heart failure.

E All children with respiratory distress should have oxygen delivery maximized.

EMQs

15–19. Match each of the following clinical presentations with the most likely diagnosis below:

15. A 15-year-old girl presents with fever and flushed skin; she has been vomiting for 2 days, and is in circulatory compromise. This is during a menstrual period with malodorous discharge. In the past, she has suffered with asthma and used to take steroid inhalers. Her heart rate 120 bpm and her C-reactive protein 240 mg/l.

16. A 6-year-old boy presents with sudden onset of loss of consciousness and generalized body stiffness. There is no history of fever or any other symptoms, and he has been very well prior to this presentation. He has been brought to the A&E Department by his father, with whom he stays at weekends. The parents separated 6 months ago, and the father has been on treatment for depression since then and was a known diabetic. The boy's pupils are semidilated, and his heart rate 65 bpm.

17. A 14-year-old boy who has previously been well has been brought to the A&E Department with sudden onset of difficulty in breathing while he was watching a local football match. He complains of chest pain. His O_2 saturation is 5 l/min, O_2 84%, respiratory rate 30/min, pulse rate 110 bpm and temperature 36.9°C. He is drowsy, his respiratory effort is poor and the air entry is reduced bilaterally.

18. An 11-day-old boy who has had had no previous perinatal problems or concerns and has been well since birth presents with sudden onset of recurrent episodes of cessation of breathing and blue discoloration, each lasting about half a minute. In between, he is unarousable. His temperature is 35°C, pulse 140 bpm and respiratory rate 40/min. On examination, he is generally hypertonic, and there is some blood oozing from his umbilical stump (the umbilical cord had come off the previous day). He was born at home.

19. A 7-month-old girl is seen after a 3-day history of loose stools and vomiting. She has been taking oral rehydration fluids and formula milk during the illness, but is vomiting. She is drowsy, with dry mucous membranes and hazy corneas. The degree of dehydration is assessed as 7%. Her skin is dough-like, and her urine osmolality is 700 mosmol with an anion gap of 15 and glucose 5.1.

Options
A Tension pneumothorax
B Meningococcal septicaemia
C Intracranial bleed
D Severe dehydration and shock
E Toxic shock syndrome
F Hypotonic dehydration
G Group B streptococcal sepsis
H Haemorrhagic disease of the newborn
I Drug overdose
J Hypertonic dehydration
K Severe acute asthma
L Meningitis

20. Match the following potentially toxic substances with an effective treatment for their toxicity below (one or more correct answers):

    (i) Tricyclic antidepressants
   (ii) Iron
  (iii) Salicylate
  (iv) Pethidine
   (v) Paracetamol
  (vi) Digoxin
 (vii) Carbon monoxide
(viii) Organophosphorus compounds

Options
A Specific antibody fragments
B Naloxone
C No specific antidote
D *N*-acetylcysteine
E Oral desferrioxamine
F Forced alkaline diuresis
G Oral methionine
H Hyperbaric oxygen
I Pralidoxime
J Intravenous desferrioxamine
K Atropine

21–25. For each of the following, choose the most appropriate diagnosis below:

21. A 3-year-old child presents with a history of loose stools, had lost some weight and had abdominal pain. His ESR is normal, and his jejunal biopsy shows total villous atrophy.

22. A 5-year-old girl presents with abdominal pain, lethargy and dysuria. Her urine shows positive nitrites and protein.

23. A 1-year-old boy is sitting on the floor and wants to rise up. He pushes his arms against the floor and uses his right arm to push his body against his legs, and stands with marked lordosis.

24. A 6-month-old child has a history of itching, crying and red skin. The skin is very dry and erythematous. No one else in the family has the same problem. He likes to play with the cat whenever near it.

25. A child presents with tachycardia, a respiratory rate of 30/min, cold peripheries and a urine specific gravity of 1025. He is very agitated and confused and wants to sleep. His blood sugar is 4.6 mmol/l and urea 13 mmol/l.

Options
A Constipation
B Moderate dehydration
C Migraine
D UTI
E Coeliac disease
F Juvenile rheumatoid arthritis
G Diabetes insipidus
H Duchenne muscular dystrophy
I Bronchiolitis
J Eczema

26–30. For each of the following, choose the most appropriate diagnosis below:

26. A 3-month-old baby boy presents with a history of heart failure. There is a systolic murmur that is not very loud on the left sternal edge at the third intercostal space. His pulses are palpable, and the first heart sound is louder. An ECG shows left ventricular hyperatrophy.

27. A 2-year-old boy presents with frequent rectal bleeding on several occasions. He is opening his bowels every second or third day, with a large amount of soft stool. He is on lactulose at 10 ml twice a day and Senokot, 5 ml every night. He has abdominal pain on a daily basis and is drinking 1 pint of fresh cows' milk per day.

28. A 13-year-old girl presents with a history of cough, temperature and lethargy. Her cough started 2 days ago with sharp chest pain on her left chest and was worse on breathing in. Her chest movement is reduced on one side, but nothing can be heard on auscultation. Her temperature is 40°C, with marked reduced air entry on the left side of her chest.

29. A 2-year-old boy presents with a history of seizures after a high temperature. He is admitted for observation after a diagnosis of a sore throat. By evening, he has become hot and more confused, and starts to have seizures for 10 minutes. He is holding his head and not able to sit up to take his milk.

30. A girl aged 12 years presents with a history of lethargy and rashes on her face, and is not able to comb her hair. Her neurological examination is normal apart from not being able to raise her hand above her head. Her temperature is 37.6°C, and she has a few small cervical (0.5 cm × 1 cm) lymph glands.

Options
A Dermatomyositis
B Cows' milk protein intolerance
C Anal fissure
D Tinea capitis
E Reactive arthritis
F Ventricular septal defect
G Transposition of the great arteries
H Fallot's tetralogy
I Meningitis
J Lobar pneumonia
K Encephalopathy
L Aortic stenosis
M Pulmonary stenosis
N Constipation
O Inflammatory bowel disease

31. **Choose for each of the following diagnoses the most appropriate investigation(s) from the list below:**

  (i) Strawberry naevus covering the left eye
  (ii) Toddler's diarrhoea
  (iii) Juvenile chronic arthritis
  (iv) Enuresis
  (v) Reflux nephropathy in a 4-year-old
  (vi) Slipped femoral epiphysis
  (vii) Thyrotoxicosis

Options
A ESR
B CRP
C DMSA
D Renal ultrasound
E Rheumatoid factors
F Antinuclear antibodies
G MSUG
H Indirect cystogram, MAG3
I Hip ultrasound
J Hip X-ray
K TSH
L FSH
M Stool for reducing substances
N T4
O Nothing
P Neck ultrasound
Q Double-stranded DNA
R LFT
S FBC
T Abdominal MRI scan
U Stool pH study
V Abdominal CT scan
W CK
X MAG3

Answers for Accident and Emergency

1. Answer: B

The majority of children attending A&E have either injuries or an infection. Most children will experience upper and lower respiratory tract infections up to six or seven times per year among the age group of 0–5 years. Family doctors can treat most of these cases, but parents want their children to be seen quickly – not the next day or even later. Primary care is under a lot of pressure with the demand of the public for treatment even for small and simple febrile illnesses. Despite the frequency of infections, injuries are the leading cause of morbidity and mortality for children between the ages of 1 and 15 years. Most of these accidents occur within the home setting, which includes the garden and its surroundings. Burns and scalds, poisonings, falls from a height, fingertip injuries and near drowning account for the vast majority of such injuries.

2. Answer: E

Pre-hospital care, i.e. family doctor and primary care, can be the link between secondary care (i.e. district general hospital) and the tertiary level (usually a teaching hospital). Two issues are important within the pre-hospital care setting: access and education.

The nursing staff usually perform triage, but it is equally acceptable for medical staff to do this.

3. Answer: A

Resuscitation

The first step in basic life support for a child found lying on the floor and not moving is 'stimulate and check responsiveness'. Second, ask for help, and then maintain the airway.

The airway can be described as open, maintainable or unmaintainable. An open airway is defined as one with no obstruction present. This includes the absence of secretions, stridor, gurgling or other noises. An open airway needs no further management, but should be kept under review. A maintainable airway is defined as one that can be kept open with simple measures such as positioning, chin lift/head tilt, the use of an oropharyngeal airway or the use of *gentle* suction. An unmaintainable airway is one that is still at risk despite these simple measures, necessitating either intubation or the creation of a surgical airway (cricothyrotomy).

The airway should be maintained by the simplest measures available. Intubation, if required, must be performed by experienced operators with skill and in a timely fashion. Any attempt taking longer than 30 seconds should be abandoned and the child oxygenated with a bag–valve–mask device, pending a second attempt.

All sick or injured children require high-flow oxygen. This should be administered using a facemask if the airway is open and maintainable. Otherwise, artificial ventilation should be established using a bag–valve–mask device.

4. Answer: A

Maintaining airways

The efficacy of breathing can be assessed only after the airway has been opened. The rate, volume and symmetry of respiration should be assessed by observation and auscultation.

Respiratory compromise can be characterized by either an increasing or a decreasing work of breathing (both of which are signs of respiratory distress or poor respiratory effort, including reduced consciousness level).

If breathing is absent or diminished, ventilation using a bag–valve–mask device should be instituted as soon as possible.

Absent breath sounds and hyper-resonance to percussion on one side should lead one to consider a pneumothorax. This should be immediately drained using a needle thoracostomy. The needle should be inserted into the midclavicular line in the second intercostal space, pending the insertion of a formal chest drain. Once inserted, the needle should be left in place until the chest drain is working properly. If signs of respiratory compromise are present, supplemental oxygen should be administered at the highest rate available.

5. Answer: B

Maintaining circulation

A central pulse should be palpated. The carotid pulse should be palpated lateral to the thyroid cartilage and medial to the sternocleidomastoid muscle in a child. In an infant, the brachial pulse should be palpated in the upper arm.

If no pulse is palpable (or the pulse is less than 60 bpm in an infant less than 1 year of age), cardiac massage should be started at a rate of 80–100 bpm. If a pulse is palpable, other evidence of circulatory embarrassment should be sought.

All children with circulatory embarrassment should have IV access established within a few minutes; otherwise, an intra-osseous needle should be inserted into the tibia or the femur up to the age of 10 years.

If signs of circulatory embarrassment or shock are present, fluid should be administered as a 20 ml/kg bolus. It does not matter at this stage whether the fluid is crystalloid or colloid, but electrolyte-poor fluids should certainly be avoided.

Blood pressure (BP) is an unreliable sign of circulatory compromise in children. Up to 40% of the circulating blood volume needs to be lost before the BP will fall. Falling BP is a late sign and indicates a failure of compensatory mechanisms to maintain perfusion to vital areas. Once the BP falls, early and urgent treatment is indicated if permanent harm is to be avoided.

6. Answer: C

Cardiac arrest

Cardiac arrest is rare in the paediatric population, but causes to consider include sudden infant death syndrome, trauma, drowning and asphyxia.

Cardiac arrest in children is primarily asystolic in nature. Occasionally, electromechanical dissociation (EMD), also known as pulseless electrical activity (PEA) or ventricular fibrillation (VF), is present. It is important to begin resuscitation, but also to consider definitive drug and fluid therapies, as indicated by the underlying rhythm.

The outcome of cardiac arrest in children is dismal, particularly when it occurs in the community. Prolonged hypoxia, hypoglycaemia and acidosis, in addition to the underlying disease process, all contribute to cell death, particularly in the myocardium and brain, making restoration of vital functions difficult. Even if cardiac function is restored, the prolonged insult to the brain usually leaves the child with permanent or profound neurological deficit.

Asystole is characterized by a pulseless, apnoeic child associated with no complexes on the cardiac monitor, but it is important to confirm this by turning up the gain on the cardiac monitor, ensuring that all the connections are made and checking that the monitor is not connected to the 'paddles' of the cardioversion equipment.

7. Answer: E

Discontinuation of resuscitation

The decision to terminate resuscitation is a difficult one. Children who have been poisoned or have drowned or who are hypothermic should have active resuscitation continued for a considerable time. In the case of an unknown cause, which could be drug overdose or poisoning, resuscitation should continue until the picture becomes clear and there has been discussion with a senior physician. This will usually occur within the intensive care setting, with continuing resuscitation during transit.

Post-traumatic cardiac arrest has a very poor prognosis, and prolonged attempts at resuscitation should be avoided. Sudden infant death syndrome should not lead to unnecessary prolonged resuscitation.

8. Answer: B

9. Answer: E

10. Answer: E

Spinal cord injury without radiological abnormality (SCIWORA)

SCIWORA is a rare finding, but has a potentially devastating outcome. Laxity of spinal ligaments in children is associated with underdevelopment of the articular facets of the vertebrae in the spinal column, allowing excessive movement to take place during severe hyperflexion/extension injuries. This may result in compression of the spinal cord. The column will return to its normal anatomy without any evidence of fracture or subluxation being present. Normal X-rays will not exclude spinal cord injury if the child is unconscious.

Note that SCIWORA is unlikely if the child moving all his/her limbs and is conscious all the time. However, in those children who have an altered level of consciousness, SCIWORA must be suspected. Full spinal column immobilization measures must be implemented if there is proof either radiologically or clinically that the spinal cord and vertebrae are intact.

The airway should be assessed and opened in the simplest way possible, and this should be carried out without moving the cervical spine.

Simple measures to immobilize the spine include the use of sandbags or other similar sized objects to immobilize the head, taping the head to a spinal board, and immobilizing the head on the shoulders using hands and arms.

11. Answer: C

Assessment

The relatively large head compared with the rest of the body makes the child more vulnerable to head injury than the adult. Most injuries are minor, with the incidence of intracranial bleeding being less in the paediatric population than the adult population.

Note that the first assessment does not need to calculate a complete coma score (e.g. the Glasgow Coma Scale): it is sufficient to document whether the child is **A**wake, responding to **V**erbal stimuli, responding to **P**ainful stimuli or **U**nresponsive (the AVPU scale). Pupillary reflexes may be documented, but at this stage they will not alter management significantly.

Once the airway, breathing and circulation have been addressed, a full secondary survey of the child should be carried out. Every part of the body will be examined both visually and by palpation. Use of a plain X-ray, ultrasound and CT will aid the diagnostic process. Minor injuries that may have been missed on the first brief survey will be detected and will lead to further treatment and investigation. Injuries that are commonly detected during the secondary survey include bleeding from the ear and nose, small pneumothoraces, gastric dilation, and minor fractures to the peripheries.

12. Answer: A

Poisoning in children

Poisoning in children is most common between the second and third years of life. Children who are poisoned usually present with minimal signs or symptoms. The role of the A&E Department is to identify the child who is at risk of either airway or circulatory collapse and to deal with these problems accordingly.

The role of gastric decontamination in this age group is controversial. The current trend is to move away from gastric lavage, which is seen as a particularly unpleasant process to inflict on children.

The role of syrup of ipecacuanha has also been challenged, as there is evidence to suggest that it will only be effective (if at all) if administered within 1 hour of ingestion of the poison.

Most children will actually drink charcoal despite its unpleasant appearance, and this is probably the method of choice for all children who require gastric decontamination.

Specific antidotes are available for only a few poisons. Staff working in A&E Departments should be familiar with these and their use.

13. Answer: D

Life-threatening infection

Life-threatening infection is relatively rare these days in the Western world, where vaccination and immunization are widely available and widespread. Diseases such as diphtheria and epiglottitis have more or less been eradicated with effective vaccination.

Meningococcaemia continues to be one of the most important life-threatening infections to appear acutely to the A&E Department. Type C has almost been eradicated in the last few years in the UK. There are still sporadic cases of type B and rarely type A in children.

Intussusception has its peak incidence in infants 3–9 months of age and is often associated with or follows gastroenteritis, Henoch–Schönlein purpura, etc.

In children aged 3 years and over, significant bacterial disease is relatively rare, but is a particular worry. Common causes include chest infection, septicaemia, urinary tract infection and orthopaedic infection.

14. Answer: E

Life-threatening infection

Children with a suspected life-threatening infection should be resuscitated and have blood taken for full blood count, urea and electrolytes, blood glucose and culture. Chest X-ray, urine culture and lumbar puncture may also be indicated. Care should be taken not to perform lumbar puncture on children who are unconscious, as this may produce herniation of the brain through the tentorium (coning), resulting in brain death. Intravenous antibiotics should not be delayed while awaiting urine or CSF samples in the acutely ill child.

Most seizure disorders presenting in status epilepticus are due to either idiopathic epilepsy or febrile seizure disorder, but rarely may be secondary to metabolic defects such as hypoglycaemia or an electrolyte disorder (although trauma may also be considered).

Comatose children are at particular risk of airway problems, so great care must be given to maintaining the airway and ventilation.

SVT is the most common underlying cardiac dysrhythmia to cause heart failure, particularly in younger age groups. SVT usually presents with irritability in babies and palpitation or a strange chest sensation in older children.

Note that all children with respiratory disease should have oxygen delivery maximized, and treatment should then be directed specifically against the underlying cause.

15–19. Answers:

15. **E:** The most likely cause is usually *Staphylococcus aureus* or a *Streptococcus* sp. Some women using tampons are at risk of this but not all. A high dose of antibiotics is recommended with high-dependency monitoring for patients with this condition, in particular for fluid balance.

16. **I:** Tricyclic antidepressants are the most likely cause. They can cause arrhythmia, especially bradycardia with cardiac arrest at any stage. Diabetic drugs will not cause this, but an open mind should be kept in all children presenting with suspected overdose.

17. **A:** This was a healthy boy who had had no problems before and suddenly developed a breathing problem. Sudden exposure to a large quantity of allergens can cause severe bronchospasms and can present like this. Reduced air entry on any side or both will raise the suspicions of a pneumothorax as well.

18. **H:** Babies who are born at home and have not received IM or oral vitamin K are at risk of developing haemorrhagic disease of the newborn. This can occur anywhere, but the usual vulnerable site is the umbilical stump.

19. **J:** It is difficult to differentiate clinically between different types of dehydration. Doughy skin is very likely associated with hypertonic dehydration.

20. Answers:

      (i) C
     (ii) E, J
    (iii) F
    (iv) B
     (v) D, G
    (vi) A
   (vii) H
  (viii) I, K

21–25. Answers:

    21. E
    22. D
    23. H
    24. J
    25. B

26–30. Answers:

    26. F
    27. B
    28. J
    29. I
    30. A

31. Answers:

      (i) O
     (ii) M, U
    (iii) A, B, E, F, Q
    (iv) O
     (v) D, H
    (vi) J
   (vii) K, N, P

Clinical Pharmacology

BOFs

1. The following are stimulant laxatives except:

   A Lactulose
   B Docusate sodium
   C Senna
   D Sodium picosulfate
   E Bisacodyl

2. The following factors increase theophylline clearance except:

   A Hyperthyroidism
   B Smoking
   C Heart failure
   D Carbamazepine
   E Charcoal-barbecued meat

3. The following drugs increase the half-life of theophylline except:

   A Ciprofloxacin
   B Propranolol
   C Cimetidine
   D Rifampicin
   E Azithromycin

4. Hypokalaemia is a well-recognized side-effect with the following diuretics except:

   A Furosemide (frusemide)
   B Polythiazides
   C Acetazolomide
   D Metolazone
   E Bendroflumethiazide (bendrofluazide)

5. The following are true about diuretics except:

   A Thiazides inhibit Na^+/Cl^- reabsorption in the early distal convoluted tubule.
   B Furosemide inhibits $Na^+/K^+/Cl^-$ cotransport in the thick ascending limb of the loop of Henle.
   C Spironolactone inhibits Na^+/K^+ exchange in the collecting duct by competing with aldosterone.
   D Acetazolomide inhibits H^+ reabsorption in the proximal tubule.
   E Mannitol increases water absorption by increasing intravascular osmolarity.

6. Regarding the use of adenosine in supraventricular tachycardia, the following are true except:

   A Adenosine is the drug of choice in children.
   B Adenosine can be given even after using a β-blocker.
   C Adenosine has a half-life of about 30 minutes.
   D Dipyridamole potentiates the action of adenosine.
   E Adenosine blocks AV nodal conduction.

7. The following β-agonists should not be used to treat an acute asthmatic attack except:

   A Salbutamol
   B Salmeterol
   C Aminophylline
   D Terbutaline
   E Theophylline

8. The mechanisms of action of β-agonists include the following except:

   A Increase insulin secretion
   B Speed plus conduction
   C Relaxation of bronchial smooth muscle
   D Antagonists at the M_2 and M_3 cholinergic receptors
   E Vasodilation in muscle

9. The following are classified as non-sedating antihistamines except:

   A Cetirizine
   B Terfenadine
   C Loratadine
   D Astemizole
   E Cyclizine

10. The following comments regarding antihistamines are true except:

    A Terfenadine has a high risk of VT.
    B Cyclizine has a marked antiemetic action.
    C Cetirizine has a high risk of VT.
    D Antihistamines should be avoided in porphyria.
    E Diphenylhydramine has some degree of sedation.

11. The following anti-asthma drug has antihistamine action:

    A Nedocromil sodium
    B Ketotifen
    C Sodium cromoglicate (cromoglycate)
    D Montelukast
    E None of the above

12. **The following drugs have a definite risk of inducing haemolysis in patients with G6PD deficiency except:**

    A Ciprofloxacin
    B Trimethoprim
    C Primaquine
    D Nitrofurantoin
    E Nalidixic acid

13. **The following comments regarding drugs and their side-effects are true except:**

    A Dapsone causes haemolysis in patients with G6PD.
    B Zidovudine can cause aplastic anaemia.
    C Prednisolone can cause thrombocytopenia.
    D Agranulocytosis can be caused by H_2 antagonists.
    E Methyldopa can cause haemolytic anaemia.

14. **The following are false regarding malaria prophylaxis except:**

    A Breastfed babies do not need it if the mother is taking prophylactic antimalarial treatment.
    B Doxycycline can be used in pregnancy.
    C Mefloquine can be used in patients with significant renal impairment.
    D Mefloquine, but not chloroquine, should be avoided where there is a history of epilepsy.
    E Prophylaxis should be started the day before travel and continued for 1–4 weeks after return, depending on the type of treatment.

15. **All of the following are true about palivizumab except:**

    A It is not contraindicated where there is a strong family history of asthma.
    B It is given once a week by intravenous infusion over 4–6 hours.
    C It is licensed for use in children with chronic lung disease and the elderly.
    D It should be started at the onset of the first respiratory infection at the beginning of the winter.
    E It is a respiratory syncytial virus (RSV) monoclonal antibody.

EMQs

16. Match each of the following drugs with one well-recognized contraindication below:

   (i) Ranitidine
   (ii) Sodium valproate
   (iii) Oxybutynin
   (iv) Gentamicin
   (v) Aspirin

   Options
   A Glaucoma
   B Lupus erythematosus
   C Intestinal obstruction
   D Severe renal impairment
   E G6PD deficiency
   F Peptic ulcer
   G Severe anaemia
   H Active liver disease

17–20. Match each of the following scenarios with the causative drug below:

   17. A 10-year-old child is diagnosed with serum sickness, immune complex glomerulonephritis and a syndrome resembling SLE.
   18. A 2-year-old child presents with a maculoerythematous rash after being given ampicillin. His grandmother died after receiving an IM injection of penicillin in her late 20s.
   19. A 5-year-old girl presents with jaundice, is pale and has fine rashes on her body. Her Coombs' test is positive, and her LFT shows a bilirubin of 270 mmol/l.
   20. Topical antibiotics were given to apply to a skin lesion on a 15-year-old girl. Her skin has become red all over the body. She has used the same antibiotics before.

   Options
   A Neomycin
   B Penicillin
   C Sulfonamides
   D Streptomycin
   E Amiodarone
   F Chlorpromazine
   G Cefotaxime
   H Methyldopa
   I Tetracycline

21–26. Which of the steroids listed below are useful in the treatment of the conditions in the following scenarios?

21. A 2-year-old is brought to A&E with a history of difficulty in breathing and audible noisy breathing, mainly on the inspiratory phase. His saturation is 90% in air. There is a marked recession, and he is using his accessory muscles.

22. A 10-year-old child is brought to hospital with a history of being unable to walk in the last 18 hours. His reflexes are absent in the left leg, and he has a very hypotonic left leg. He is rushed to have a MRI scan, which shows increased density in the white matter, mainly around the anterior horns on the right side. He suffered from an URTI 2 weeks ago.

23. A 3-year-old girl presents with a 3-hour history of flaring rashes over her body. It looks like an urticarial rash. It is itchy, and she says that her throat is hurting her.

24. A known asthmatic is admitted to hospital with exacerbation of his asthma. He had 10 puffs of salbutamol via a spacer, which is repeated at hourly intervals.

25. A 1-year-old boy presents with history of a flared rash over his face and neck. This has been going on since he was 3 months old. He has tested allergic to cows' milk and egg white.

26. A known congenital adrenal hyperplasia patient is admitted with a history of excessive vomiting. She is on 5 mg of hydrocortisone three times a day. Her sodium is high and her potassium low. She is resuscitated with fluids and drugs.

Options
A   Beclometasone (beclomethasone)
B   Hydrocortisone
C   Hydrocortisone 1–2%
D   Prednisolone
E   Fludrocortisone
F   Methylprednisolone
G   Dexamethasone
H   Aldosterone

27–30. For each of the following scenarios, match the appropriate drugs of choice for treatment:

27. A 6-month-old baby boy presents with a history of lethargy, not feeding, sweating and looking very anxious. His heart rate is above 260 bpm. His ECG shows a narrow complex with the presence of a P-wave.

28. A 9-month-old girl presents with a history of sweating and not always being able to finish her bottle. She is below the third centile and had an URTI 2 days ago. Her liver is 4 cm large, and her heart rate 110 bpm.

29. An 11-month-old boy is diagnosed as having heart failure secondary to cardiomyopathy. He had a virus-like illness 2 weeks ago. He is not known to have had any problems prior to this, and there is no family history of any illnesses.

30. A 9-year-old girl presents with a history of losing weight, tachycardia, protuberant eyes, much sweating, a very short temper and hyperactivity. Her T_4 is 200 nmol/l.

Options
A Digoxin
B Propanolol
C Verapamil
D Adenosine
E Amiodarone
F Furosemide (frusemide)
G Captopril
H Dobutamine
I Adrenaline
J Flecainide
K Calcium chloride
L Magnesium
M Isoprenaline
N Lidocaine (lignocaine)

31. Match each of the following drugs with three of their well-recognized side-effects below:

 (i) Ketamine
 (ii) Carbamazepine
(iii) Phenytoin
(iv) Oxybutynin
 (v) Propanolol
(vi) Methylphenidate

Options
A Amnesia
B Facial flushing
C Hallucinations
D Bronchospasm
E Thrombocytopenia
F Arrhythmias
G Hypotension
H Tics
I Hypertension
J Respiratory depression
K Constipation
L Heart failure
M Transient psychosis
N Hepatitis

Answers for Clinical Pharmacology

1. Answer: A

Laxatives

Macrogols and lactulose are osmotic laxatives. They act by retaining fluid in the bowel by osmosis. Lactulose passes through the small intestine unchanged but in the colon is broken down by carbohydrate-fermenting bacteria to produce unabsorbed organic anions that retain fluid in the gut lumen and also make the colon contents more acidic. An effect is usually produced after 2–3 days. Lactulose is very effective in treating hepatic encephalopathy because of its action.

Senna is one of many stimulants, which also include bisacodyl, glycerol suppositories and phosphates. Senna is hydrolysed by colonic bacteria to the active principles sennasoid A and sennasoid B, which enhance the normal response of the colon to stimuli. It is important to combine senna with a high-bulk diet to get normal physiological stimuli. It will take 8 hours to produce an effect.

Stimulant laxatives act by increasing intestinal motility and so may cause abdominal cramps. Their prolonged use, which may be necessary in some cases, may cause hypokalaemia and an atonic non-functional colon.

Lubricants such as docusate sodium (dioctyl sodium sulfosuccinate) and liquid paraffin act by softening or lubricating the faeces.

Bulk laxatives such as plant fibres (bran) are resistant to digestion in the intestine, increase the bulk of stool and reduce the bowel transient time due to the ability of fibre to absorb water and swell.

2. Answer: C

3. Answer: D

Theophylline and its derivatives

Factors that increase theophylline clearance	Factors that decrease theophylline clearance
Marijuana	Congestive cardiac failure
Smoking	Neonates
High-protein, low-carbohydrate diet	Pneumonia
Hyperthyroidism	Old age
Ethanol	Antifungals
Rifampicin	Cimetidine
Phenytoin	Ciprofloxacin
Carbamazepine	Chloramphenicol
Charcoal-barbecued meat	Erythromycin and other macrolides
	Influenza vaccine and interferon
	Propranolol
	Ketoconazole
	Hepatic diseases
	Contraceptives

Theophylline is a β_2 agonist and causes bronchiodilation by increasing intracellular cAMP. It is one of the phosphodiesterase inhibitors used in the treatment of asthma. There are IV and oral preparations. Theophylline relaxes airway smooth muscle and inhibits the release of mediators from mast cells. It is also a potent antagonist of adenosine by blocking A_2 receptors. It also has an anti-inflammatory activity on T lymphocytes by reducing release of platelet-activating factors. Theophylline also reduces calcium entry via receptor-operated channels. It is a central respiratory stimulant and increases the force of contraction of respiratory muscles. Therapeutic drug monitoring can be performed. The side-effects of theophylline include gastrointestinal disturbances, vasodilation, arrhythmias, seizures and sleep disturbances.

4. Answer: C

5. Answer: D

Diuretics

Furosemide (frusemide) is a loop diuretic and is mainly used in heart failure and in patients with chronic renal failure who are suffering from fluid overload and/or hypertension. It inhibits $Na^+/K^+/Cl^-$ cotransport in the thick ascending limb of the loop of Henle. It is bound to plasma proteins and is eliminated via the kidneys.

The side-effects of furosemide include acute renal failure, hyperuricaemia and gout, hypokalaemia, hypomagnesaemia, carbohydrate intolerance, ototoxicity, idiosyncratic blood dyscrasias, and metabolic acidosis. It increases the nephrotoxicity of cephaloridine, but most recent cephalosporins show less nephrotoxicity. Indomethacin inhibits prostaglandin biosynthesis and opposes the diuretic effect of loop diuretics, inhibiting secretion into the tubule.

Thiazides are also used frequently. These include bendroflumethiazide (bendrofluazide), hydrochlorothiazide and metolazone. They are used in the treatment of hypertension, cardiac failure, resistant oedema and diabetes insipidus and in the prevention of stones. They decrease Na^+/Cl^- reabsorption in the early part of the distal convoluted tubule and so increase the excretion of sodium, water and chloride. In addition, thiazides relax smooth muscles, which is why they are used in the treatment of hypertension. Their side-effects include impotence, impairment of glucose tolerance, hyperuricaemia, hyponatraemia, hypokalaemia, hypomagnesaemia and allergy. They reduce lithium excretion as well as that of other diuretics. When treating certain conditions, thiazides are usefully combined with various other drugs, such as β-adrenoreceptor antagonists, α_1-adrenoreceptor antagonists and converting-enzyme inhibitors.

Spironolactone, amiloride and triamterene are potassium-sparing diuretics. They inhibit Na^+/K^+ exchange in the collecting duct either by competing with aldosterone (spironolactone) or non-competitively (amiloride and triamterene). They are not potent diuretics, but, combined with other diuretics such as thiazide and loop diuretics, they work much better and there are fewer side-effects from either. The main side-effect is hyperkalaemia.

Acetazolamide is a carbonic anhydrase inhibitor. It inhibits bicarbonate reabsorption in the proximal tubule and may cause hypokalaemia and acidosis. It is used for many conditions, including intracranial hypertension, motion sickness, renal tubular acidosis and glaucoma, and is also used as an anticonvulsant. Another carbonic anhydrase inhibitor, dorzolamide, is used topically for glaucoma.

Mannitol is an osmotic diuretic and is used in patients with incipient acute renal failure, acutely low intracranial pressure and low intraocular pressure. Mannitol increases water absorption by increasing intravascular osmolarity.

6. Answer: C

Adenosine

Adenosine has a short half-life of 8–10 seconds, but this is prolonged in patients taking dipyridamole. Most of its side-effects are short-lived. Asthma is a contraindication for using adenosine. Verapamil may be preferred in asthmatic patients. Adenosine is used to terminate SVT and in regular narrow complex tachycardia if one is not sure of SVT. It has no effect on VT. It also contracts bronchial smooth muscle and relaxes vascular smooth muscle. It inhibits platelet aggregation via A_2 receptors. The side-effects of adenosine include chest pain, flushing, dizziness, shortness of breath and nausea. It should be used with care in WPW syndrome and is contraindicated in heart block unless a pacemaker is in place.

7. Answer: B

8. Answer: D

β-agonists

These cause bronchiodilation by increasing intracellular cAMP. The short-acting agents are used in the treatment of acute asthma attacks. The long-acting agents are used regularly once or twice a day, although they are no good for acute attacks. The common side-effects of β-agonists are tremors, tachycardia, hypokalaemia, vasodilation and hyperglycaemia.

Eformetrol and salmeterol are long-acting β-agonists and should be used in prophylaxis, including for nocturnal and exercise-induced asthma. Their mechanisms of action are many, and some of these agents will cause adverse effects.

β-agonists relax the bronchial smooth muscles, inhibit the release of inflammatory mediators, increase mucociliary clearance, relax uterine smooth muscle, increase heart rate, cause muscle tremors, vasodilation in muscles and hypokalaemia via redistribution of potassium into cells, raise free fatty acid concentrations, and increase insulin excretion (but they also increase glycogenolysis).

9. Answer: E

10. Answer: C

11. Answer: B

Antihistamines (H$_1$-receptor antagonists)

These are used in the treatment of hypersensitivity and are effective in urticaria, hayfever and anaphylactic shock. They are not useful in the treatment of asthma. Antihistamines are also used to prevent motion sickness, in treating the common cold and sinusitis, and in cough mixtures. They block oedema and vascular responses to histamine. They have an antiemetic effect. The major side-effects include sedation (with some), psychomotor impairment, nausea, photosensitive rashes, dry mouth, blurred vision and (in the case of terfenadine and astemizole) prolongation of the QT interval when given with other drugs that block the metabolism of the antihistamine, such as ketoconazole and erythromycin (this also happens with overdoses). Antihistamines should be avoided in porphyria and Ward–Romano syndrome.

Sedating antihistamines	*Non-sedating antihistamines*
All are first-generation	All are second-generation
All have a short half-life	All have a long half-life
Promethazine	Acrivastine (no risk of VT)
Diphenhydramine	Terfenadine (high risk of VT)
Chlorpheniramine	Fexofenadine (no risk of VT)
Cyclizine	Astemizole (high risk of VT)
Triprolidine	Cetirizine (no risk of VT)
	Loratidine (no risk of VT)

12. Answer: B

13. Answer: C

Trimethoprim is not included in the BNF in the lists of drugs that have definite or possible risks of inducing haemolysis in patients with G6PD deficiency. Co-trimoxazole (because it contains a sulfonamide) has a definite risk, as do other substances, including fava beans, dapsone, methylene blue and sulphonamides. Drugs that do not cause haemolysis in G6PD patients include aspirin, chloroquine, probenacid, quinidine and quinine.

Cancer chemotherapy can cause bone marrow suppression. Aplastic anaemia can be caused by chloramphenicol, indometacin (indomethacin) and carbimazole. Drugs that can cause agranulocytosis are carbamezapine, propylthiouracil, chlorpromazine, and clozapine. Drugs that cause thrombocytopaenia are heparin, azathioprine, quinidine and thiazides. Drugs that cause haemolytic anaemia include methyldopa and β-lactams (penicillin and cephalosporins).

14. Answer: C

Malaria prophylaxis

Breastfed babies will require prophylaxis even if the mother is taking prophylactic antimalarial treatment. The secretion of antimalarial drugs into the milk is too variable to be reliable.

Note that the use of mefloquine is considered appropriate in patients with significant renal impairment, and dose reduction is not necessary.

Doxycycline can also be used in renal impairment, but is contraindicated in pregnancy.

Both mefloquine and chloroquine are unsuitable where there is a history of epilepsy.

Prophylaxis should be started at least 1 week before travel (1–2 days for Malarone (proguanil plus atovaquone)) and continued for 4 weeks after return (1 week for Malarone).

15. Answer: B

Palivizumab (Synagis)

Palivizumab is a monoclonal antibody licensed for monthly use to prevent RSV infections in infants who were born at 35 weeks of gestation or less and are still under 6 months of age at the start of the RSV season and children less than 2 years old who have received treatment for bronchopulmonary dysplasia within the last 6 months.

The course should be started before the start of the RSV season.

It is given by intramuscular injection and is contraindicated if there has been hypersensitivity to human monoclonal antibodies.

16. Answers:

    (i) E
    (ii) H
   (iii) A
   (iv) D
    (v) F

17–20. Answers:

17. B, C, D
18. B, G
19. B, G, H
20. A, B

Types of drug allergies

Type I reaction: This is usually caused by β-lactams such as penicillin and cephalosporins. It is due to production of IgE antibodies. The antigen–antibody reaction on the surface of mast cells produces a reaction.

Type II reaction: This is due to antibodies of class IgG and IgM activating complement and causing cell lysis. Penicillin, cephalosporins and methyldopa will cause haemolytic anaemia with a positive Coombs' test.

Type III reaction: A circulating immune complex can produce severe allergic reactions, including serum sickness, immune complex glomerulonephritis and a syndrome resembling SLE. Penicillin, streptomycin, sulfonamides and propylthiouracil will cause this reaction.

Type IV reaction: A delayed hypersensitivity reaction looks like contact dermatitis following the application of topical antibiotics such as neomycin and penicillin.

21–26. Answers:

21. A, G: beclometasone (Pulmicort) nebulized and/or dexamethasone oral
22. F: methylprednisolone IV
23. B: hydrocortisone IV
24. D: prednisolone oral
25. C: hydrocortisone 1–2% topical
26. B, E: hydrocortisone IV and fludrocortisone

Steroids

Note that 5 mg prednisolone = 20 mg hydrocortisone = 6 mg deflazacort = 0.75 μg dexamethasone = 4 mg methylprednisolone.

Patients receiving oral or parenteral corticosteroids are at an increased risk of severe chickenpox unless they have had chickenpox in the past or they are receiving the treatment as replacement therapy. VZIG is indicated for patients who are on steroids at exposure and for those who have received steroids (in immunosuppressive doses) within the previous 3 months. It should be given within 3 days (and not later than 10 days) of exposure. Steroids should not be stopped in confirmed cases of chickenpox, and in fact the dose may need to be increased. Inhaled, rectal and topical steroids are less likely to be associated with an increased risk.

Side-effects are many with the chronic use of steroids – e.g. Cushing's syndrome, hypertension, hyperglycaemia, immunodeficiency, osteoporosis, growth failure, peptic ulceration, fluid and electrolyte imbalance, anxiety, elation, insomnia, depression and psychosis, subcapsular cataracts, proximal myopathy, teratogenicity, and aseptic necrosis of bones.

27–30. Answers:

> **27.** D, J: adenosine IV and flecainide as maintenance
> **28.** F, G: furosemide IV to start with, then oral, captopril oral and monitor
> **29.** E, F: amiodarone oral and furosemide oral, and follow-up regularly
> **30.** B

Heart failure and arrhythmias

These are usually associated with congenital or valvular heart disease. Cardiomyopathy and hypertension are other causes, but are rare in children. Activation of the sympathetic and renin–angiotensin systems may have an adverse effect. Treatment can be specific, such as valve replacement or correction of congenital heart abnormalities. Preload is reduced by diuretics, nitrites and ACE inhibitors (e.g. captopril). Afterload is reduced by ACE inhibitors and hydralazine. Contractility is increased by digoxin and dobutamine. Heart rate is slowed by digoxin, as in atrial fibrillation, which is rare in children.

Flecainide slows dissociation from Na^+ channel and is used as maintenance in SVT by prolonging His–Purkinje conduction. Lidocaine is used in the treatment of VT and fibrillation. β-adrenoceptor antagonists are used in sinus tachycardia in anxious patients, SVT that follows emotion or anxiety, and tachycardia associated with thyrotoxicosis. Amiodarone is used in the treatment of SVT, VT and fibrillation.

31. Answers:

> **(i)** C, I, M
> **(ii)** E, K, N
> **(iii)** E, F, G, J
> **(iv)** B, C, F, K
> **(v)** D, G, L
> **(vi)** E, H, I

Genetics

BOFs

1. The following are true about autosomal recessive disorders except:

   A They can only be inherited through non-sex chromosomes.
   B *Both* genes of a pair must be abnormal to produce disease.
   C There is a 25% chance of each child inheriting one abnormal gene and becoming a carrier.
   D If both parents are carriers, then one child is not a carrier and does not have the disease.
   E Each child will have a 1 in 4 chance of inheriting the disorder.

2. All of the following are true about X-linked recessive disorders except:

   A Half of the daughters will have the affected gene.
   B The disease only manifests in half of the sons.
   C Half of the sons do not have the gene and cannot pass it on.
   D There is no male-to-male transmission.
   E They are not compatible with life.

3. The following diseases are inherited in an autosomal dominant manner except:

   A Marfan's syndrome
   B Osteosclerosis
   C Neurofibromatosis
   D Alpers' syndrome
   E Polycystic kidney diseases

4. The following are autosomal disorders except:

   A Sickle cell anaemia
   B Spinal muscular dystrophy
   C Galactosaemia
   D Cystic fibrosis
   E Tay–Sachs disease

5. The following are X-linked recessive genetic disorders except:

   A Haemophilia A
   B Incontinentia pigmenti
   C Wiskott–Aldrich syndrome
   D Red–green colour blindness
   E Progressive spinal muscular dystrophy

6. All of the following are true about syndromes and chromosomal abnormalities except:

   A Cri-du-chat syndrome: 5p15.2–15.3 deletion
   B Edwards' syndrome: trisomy 13
   C Williams' syndrome: 7q11.23 deletion
   D Angelman's syndrome: 15q11–13 deletion (maternal)
   E Alagille's syndrome: 20p12.1–11.23

7. All of the following are classified as chromosomal breakage syndromes except:

   A Ataxia telangiectasia
   B Alkaptonuria
   C Bloom's syndrome
   D Fanconi's anaemia
   E Xeroderma pigmentosum

8. The following syndromes can be included in the differential diagnosis of asphyxiating thoracic dystrophy (Jeune's syndrome) except:

   A Achondroplasia
   B Hypophosphatasia
   C Ellis–van Creveld syndrome
   D Osteogenesis imperfecta
   E Thanatophoric dysplasia

9. The following statements are true about Ehlers–Danlos syndrome except:

   A Skin hyperextensibility
   B Joint hypermobility and excessive dislocations
   C Blue sclera
   D Tissue fragility
   E Poor wound healing

10. The following factors contribute to early death in Down's syndrome except:

   A Congenital heart disease
   B Oesophageal atresia
   C Premature ageing
   D Hirschsprung's disease
   E Leukaemia

EMQs

11–15. Choose from the following descriptions the most appropriate diagnosis from the list below:

11. A 9-year-old girl with hypoplasia of her auricles, contruncal cardiac anomalies that corrected but were still cyanotic from time to time, a cleft palate that repaired, short stature and cellular immune problems.

12. A 13-year-old boy, above the 99th centile for height, with gynaecomastia and small testes. The karyotype is 47XXY.

13. A 7-year-old girl who is on the 0.2 centile for height, with webbed neck, widely spaced nipples, underdeveloped gonads and a karyotype showing 45X.

14. A 12-year-old boy with learning difficulties and seizures. A large jaw, macro-orchidism and large prominent ears are the main features found on examination. The gene is located on the distal arm of chromosome X at Xq27.3.

15. A 6-year-old boy with round face, thick upper lip and full cheeks. There are stellate patterns in the iris and strabismus, with supravalvular aortic arch stenosis on echocardiography. He is described as a happy child and gets on well with others.

Options
A Fragile X syndrome
B Down's syndrome
C Alagille's syndrome
D Williams' syndrome
E Prader–Willi syndrome
F Klinefelter's syndrome
G DiGeorge veloacardiofacial syndrome ('Catch 22')
H Laurence–Moon–Biedl syndrome
I Smith–Magenis syndrome
J Cri-du-chat syndrome
K Cornelia de Lange syndrome
L Turner's syndrome

Answers for Genetics

I. Answer: C

Autosomal recessive disorders

There is a 50% chance of each child inheriting one abnormal gene and becoming a carrier. If it is assumed that 4 children are produced and both parents are carriers then the risk for the offspring will be as follows:

- I child with 2 normal chromosomes will be normal
- 2 children with I normal and I abnormal chromosome will be carriers, but not have the disease
- I child with 2 abnormal chromosomes will have the disease

This mean that *each* child has a I in 4 chance of inheriting the disorder and a 50 : 50 chance of being a carrier.

2. Answer: E

X-linked recessive disorders

Half of the daughters have the gene and can pass it to the next generation. The other half do not have the gene, and therefore cannot pass it on. Half of the sons do not have the gene, and cannot pass it on. The other half of the sons have inherited the gene and will express the trait or disorder. The majority of these disorders are compatible with life, with intense management and support.

3. Answer: D

4. Answer: C

Autosomal disorders

Alpers' syndrome is inherited as an autosomal recessive disorder, as are thalassaemia, some muscular dystrophies, Usher's syndrome, the majority of inborn errors of metabolism and rare cases of polycystic kidney disease. Tuberous sclerosis, achondroplasia and most inherited cases of polycystic kidney disease are inherited as autosomal dominant disorders. Galactosaemia is an X-linked genetic disorder.

5. Answer: B

X-linked disorders

Galactosaemia, Becker muscular dystrophy, Duchene muscular dystrophy, fragile X syndrome and X-linked agammaglobulinaemia are inherited as X-linked recessive disorders. Incontinentia pigmenti and Coffen's syndrome are X-linked dominant.

6. Answer: B

Chromosomal abnormalities

Edwards' syndrome is trisomy 18 (trisomy 13 is Patau's syndrome). *Paternal* deletion of 15q11–13 results in Prader–Willi syndrome rather than Angelman's syndrome. Rubinstein–Taybi syndrome is associated with deletion of 16p13.3, Miller–Diecker lissencephaly with deletion of 17p13.3, Smith–Magenis syndrome with deletion of 17p11.2 and DiGeorge velocardiofacial syndrome ('Catch 22') with deletion at 22q11.21–11.23.

7. Answer: B

Chromosomal breakage syndromes

These are a group of genetic disorders, all of which are transmitted in an autosomal recessive manner. When cells are cultured from infected individuals, these cells will demonstrate variable rates of chromosomal breakage or instability, leading to chromosomal rearrangements. These disorders are characterized by a defect in DNA repair mechanisms or by genomic instability, and patients show an increased predisposition to cancer. All patients are very sensitive to ultraviolet (UV) radiation. Ataxia telangiectasia also shows hypersensitivity to ionizing radiation. These are very rare disorders and are often lethal.

8. Answer: C

Asphyxiating thoracic dystrophy (Jeune's syndrome)

This is a potentially lethal congenital dwarfism, usually inherited in an autosomal recessive manner and very rare. It is characterized by typical skeletal dysplasias, such as a narrow thorax and micromelia, with respiratory and renal manifestations. The respiratory manifestations vary widely from respiratory failure and infantile death to a latent phenotype without respiratory symptoms. Other conditions to be included in the differential diagnosis are achondrogenesis and cartilage–hair hypoplasia.

9. Answer: C

Ehlers–Danlos syndrome (EDS)

This inherited disorder can be AR, AD or X-linked. It comprises a group of conditions sharing a common reduction in the tensile strength of skin, joints and other tissues. Individuals with EDS demonstrate connective tissue abnormalities as a result of defects in the inherent strength, elasticity, integrity and healing properties of the tissues. EDS is characterized by aberrant functioning of the extracellular connective tissue matrix.

10. Answer: C

Down's syndrome

Other factors include duodenal atresia, tracheo-esophageal fistula and congenital brain abnormalities. Death in later life is due to premature ageing. About 75% of concepti with trisomy 21 die in embryonic or fetal life. The survival rate in infants up to 1 year of age is 85%, and 50% can be expected to live longer than 50 years. The presence of congenital heart disease is the most significant factor that determines survival. Morbidity is high due to infection as a result of immune system problems. Large tonsils and adenoids, lingual tonsils, choanal stenosis, or large tongue can obstruct the upper airway. Serous otitis media, alveolar hypoventilation, arterial hypoxaemia, cerebral hypoxia, and development of pulmonary artery hypertension with resulting cor pulmonale and heart failure all result from airway obstructions and heart problems. Atlantoaxial and atlanto-occipital instability may result in irreversible spinal cord damage if not recognized early enough, and any surgical procedures requiring general anaesthesia should be performed very carefully. Learning difficulties and visual and hearing problems can be expected in the majority of these children. Regular thyroid function checks will prevent further developmental delay.

11. Answer: G

DiGeorge velocardiofacial syndrome ('Catch 22')

These children also have behavioural problems, thymus aplasia and parathyroid gains.

12. Answer: F

Klinefelter's syndrome

The phenotype is male with 47XXY, with delayed development of secondary sexual character. They usually have azoospermia and are infertile.

13. Answer: L

Turner's syndrome

This is characterized by loss of all or part of the sex chromosome. Half of affected individuals are 45X on lymphocyte studies, and the other half will have a variety of abnormalities of one of their sex chromosomes. The phenotypes are female, and other features include a wide carrying angle, alopecia, and developmental delay with infertility.

14. Answer: A

Fragile X syndrome

This is the most common form of mental retardation in males. The fragile site (*FRAXA*) only becomes visible in chromosome studies when a special culture technique is applied. They also have stereotyped behaviour and speech. Females affected with fragile X may show degrees of mental retardation.

15. Answer: D

Williams' syndrome

This may show other cardiac malformations. Mental retardation and learning difficulties are, to a certain degree, associated with all affected individuals. They have a very friendly personality.

Immunology

BOFs

1. **The following are true about chronic granulomatous disease except:**

   A It is characterized by abnormalities of NADPH oxidase.
   B It is inherited in an X-linked manner.
   C Carrier status can be determined by NBT-positive cells.
   D Prenatal diagnosis can be made on tissue obtained by chorionic villus sampling in the first trimester.
   E It is characterized by diffuse granulomata in respiratory, gastro-intestinal or urogenital tracts.

2. **IgG subclass deficiency is associated with the following except:**

   A IgG2 is associated with low IgA.
   B IgG2 is associated with poor antibody responses to polysaccharide antigens.
   C It is usually a permanent problem.
   D Severe IgG2 deficiency may lead to bronchiectasis.
   E Prophylactic antibiotics can be used to prevent severe infections.

3. **The following are true with regard to Wiskott–Aldrich syndrome except:**

   A It is inherited as an autosomal dominant disorder.
   B It is associated with microthrombocytopenia, eczema and immunodeficiency.
   C Intrinsic abnormalities of B-cell function are a common feature.
   D Low levels of IgM and increased levels of IgA, IgD and IgE can found.
   E Splenectomy is usually effective in increasing platelet numbers.

4. **The following are primary immune deficiency diseases except:**

   A Purine nucleoside phosphorylase
   B Adenosine deaminase
   C Severe combined immune deficiency
   D Wiskott–Aldrich syndrome
   E Autoimmune deficiency syndrome

5. The presentation of a child with severe combined immune deficiency can be as follows except:

   A Failure to thrive
   B Pneumonitis
   C Diarrhoea
   D Eczema
   E Recurrent thrush

6. Transient hypogammaglobulinaemia in infants is associated with the following except:

   A Antibody responses to vaccines may be poor initially, but responses to boosters are normal.
   B The lymphocyte subpopulation is abnormal.
   C All immunoglobulins are low.
   D It may cause deafness.
   E Prophylactic antibiotics can be used in these cases.

7. In X-linked agammaglobulinaemia all of the following are true except:

   A B cells are absent.
   B It is X-linked recessive and is caused by defects in a gene located at Xq22.
   C The most common organisms causing infection are *Staphylococcus aureus* and *Neisseria meningitidis*.
   D Infection with *Giardia lamblia* is not uncommon.
   E Neutropenia may be present, particularly during severe infections.

8. The following are causes of neutropenia except:

   A Shwachman–Diamond syndrome
   B Glycogen storage disease type 1b
   C Dyskeratosis congenita
   D DiGeorge syndrome
   E Chediak–Higashi syndrome

9. The following are T-cell disorders except:

   A Omenn's syndrome
   B DiGeorge syndrome
   C Shwachman–Diamond syndrome
   D Wiskott–Aldrich syndrome
   E Severe combined immune deficiency

10. **The following statements are true about the complement systems except:**

    A Deficiencies in the classical pathway (C1, C4 and C2) are associated with immune complex diseases.

    B Deficiencies in the alternative pathway (properdin, factor B and factor D) are associated with severe fulminant pyogenic neisserial infections.

    C Deficiencies in C3, factor H and factor I predispose to pyogenic bacterial infections.

    D Deficiencies in the terminal pathway (C5–C9) predispose to neisserial and bacterial infections.

    E Complement system activated by cellular immunity.

EMQs

11–15. **Chose from the following scenarios the most likely diagnosis from the list below:**

11. A 10-month-old boy presents with second lobar pneumonia over the last 3 months. The level of all immunoglobulins is low, and the tonsils are hypoplastic as are the adenoids. Peripheral blood B lymphocytes are absent.

12. A 7-month-old girl presents with cough and high temperature. Chest X-ray shows interstitial pneumonitis. She is tested for HIV, CF and Ig levels, which are all normal. Bronchoscopy is performed and *Pneumocystis carinii* is isolated. CD3$^+$ T lymphocytes are decreased and thymic hypoplasia is noticed on chest CT scan.

13. A 12-month-old boy presents with frequent bacterial and viral infection. T-cell function is low. The child shows failure to thrive, oral candidiasis, and skin infections on his buttocks and legs. The full blood count shows neutropenia, eosinophilia and lymphopenia. Serum IgG is normal, with low IgA. IgE is markedly elevated, as is IgD.

14. A 2-year-old child presents with a history of recurrent UTI and chest infection. The mother recalls that umbilical cord separation occurred at the age of 3 weeks. He suffered from a skin infection, which required admission for IV antibiotics for 2 weeks and plastic surgery on his left shoulder. Neutrophil and monocyte adherence, aggregation and chemotaxis, and phagocytosis demonstrate abnormalities. Autoantibodies and response to vaccination are normal.

15. A 6-year-old girl has a bone marrow transplant for ALL. She presents with erythroderma, abnormal liver function and diarrhoea 3 weeks after the transplant.

A   Chronic graft-versus-host disease
B   Chronic granulomatous disease
C   Chediak–Higashi syndrome
D   X-linked agammaglobulinaemia
E   Leukocyte adhesion deficiency
F   Severe combined immune deficiency
G   IgG subclass deficiency
H   Autoimmune deficiency syndrome
I   Acute graft-versus-host disease
J   Ataxia telangiectasia
K   Purine nucleoside deficiency
L   DiGeorge syndrome
M   Common variable immunodeficiency

Answers for Immunology

1. Answer: C

Chronic granulomatous disease (CGD)

CGD is characterized by abnormalities of NADPH oxidase. Effective neutrophil phagocytosis requires activation of NADPH-dependent oxidase. This is most abundant in phagocytic cells, particularly neutrophils, eosinophils and cells of the monocyte/macrophage lineage. NADPH oxidase catalyses the formation of superoxide, which is a precursor for the generation of potent oxidant compounds, by transmembrane passage of electrons from NADPH to molecular O_2. About one-third of patients with CGD have inherited it in an autosomal recessive manner. Autosomal recessive CGD has been shown to be due to abnormalities in $p47^{phox}$, $p67^{phox}$ and $p22^{phox}$. The X-linked form is due to abnormalities in $gp91^{phox}$. Both $p22^{phox}$ and $gp91^{phox}$ are missing in cells derived from most CGD patients with a molecular lesion of either subunit, indicating that mutual interaction is necessary for assembly of the mature complex. Individuals with X-linked disease are said to have a more severe clinical phenotype and increased mortality.

Recurrent unusual lymphadenitis, hepatic abscesses, osteomyelitis at multiple sites, a family history of recurrent infection, or unusual infection can be the presentation of CGD or make the diagnosis of CGD highly suspicious. Catalase-positive organisms (e.g. *Staphylococcus aureus*) are usually the causative organisms.

The nitroblue tetrazolin dye test (NBT) will help in diagnosing CGD, and mixed NBT-positive and NBT-negative cells will help in identifying carriers.

A bone marrow transplant is curative for this condition.

2. Answer: C

IgG subclass deficiency

This is a very rare condition that sometimes may be responsible for primary severe immune deficiency. Children usually present with upper respiratory tract infection. It can be familial, and repeated infection may cause bronchiectasis. It usually resolves spontaneously, and immunoglobulin is not needed except in cases with severe recurrent infection. Prophylactic azithromycin or Augmentin is advisable. No routine blood tests or chest X-rays are needed.

3. Answer: A

Wiskott–Aldrich syndrome (WAS)

This is inherited as an X-linked recessive disease and is a rare condition. It is usually characterized by immune dysregulation (immune deficiency, eczema or autoimmunity) and microthrombocytopenia. Patients with WAS are compromised immunologically, and are susceptible to pyogenic, viral and opportunistic infections. They also develop eczema, a spectrum of autoimmune phenomena and lymphoproliferative disease. The platelets are small, and it can present with minor bruising as well as life-threatening GIT or intracranial bleeding. The T cells are progressively reduced in number and function during childhood, which leads to both restricted defects in proliferative responses of $WASp^{-/-}$ T cells and impaired delayed-type hypersensitivity (DTH) responses. Deficient antibody responses to polysaccharide (PS) antigens in particular, and low or absent levels of isohaemagglutinins, suggest that there are also intrinsic abnormalities of B-cell function. WAS is associated with low levels of IgM and increased levels of IgA, IgD and IgE. Gene mutations are expected with classic WAS. Using prophylactic antibiotics and immunoglobulin for infection is the conventional therapy. Splenectomy is usually effective in increasing platelet numbers and reducing bleeding complications, but also increases the risk of infection. Stem cell transplantation is curative and gene therapy may help in the future. Major complications associated with WAS include autoimmune phenomena, including haematological cytopenias, small- and large-vessel vasculitis, lymphoproliferative disease, and lymphoma.

4. Answer: E

Primary immune deficiencies

Others include CGD, agammaglobulinaemia, cytokine defects and IgG subclass deficiency.

5. Answer: D

Severe combined immune deficiency

This has a heterogeneous clinical and immunological phenotype, and in many cases the abnormalities are unknown. It can arise from a number of defined molecular defects. Patients can present with failure to thrive, diarrhoea and recurrent opportunistic infections, which can be very severe. Recurrent thrush and skin rashes from viral infections also occur. Interstitial pneumonitis due to opportunistic infections is commonly seen. *Pneumocystis carinii*, respiratory syncytial virus, cytomegalovirus, adenovirus, influenza and parainfluenza are all responsible for respiratory infections. If BCG is given at birth to these children, they may develop BCG infection. This may have severe consequences, with widespread disease in the lungs, liver, spleen and GIT. Bacterial and fungal pneumonias have also been described, and prognosis is poor if effective measures are not taken early. A bone marrow transplant is the only curative procedure in these cases, and early referral should be made to avoid death. Enzyme replacement therapy and gene therapy can be used in other types of SCID.

6. Answer: B

Transient hypogammaglobulinaemia in infancy

This may be due to delayed maturation of normal immunoglobulin production. In most cases, complete resolution occurs, and only a small group may progress to common variable immunodeficiency. It can present as recurrent upper respiratory infection and sometimes as severe infection. Bronchiectasis and deafness may occur as a result of severe infection and may be recurrent. The majority of cases resolve, although a few may need immunoglobulins or prophylactic antibiotics. The lymphocyte subpopulation is normal, and all immunoglobulin levels are low.

7. Answer: C

X-linked agammaglobulinaemia (XLA)

This affects males, with a repeated history of bacterial infection. It usually occurs after 6 months of age and before 2 years of age. Mild forms may present later in childhood, or even in adolescence or early adulthood. The most frequent sites of infection are otitis, sinusitis and pneumonia, and the most common organisms are *Haemophilus influenzae* and *Streptococcus pneumoniae*. Non-infectious manifestations (e.g. arthritis) are unusual in XLA, but have been described. *Pneumocystis carinii* pneumonia is very rare, but infection with *Giardia lamblia* is not uncommon. Neutropenia may be present during severe infections, but not other times.

All isotypes of immunoglobulins are absent or very low. Circulating mature B cells are absent, as are specific antibodies. T cells are normal. Children with XLA will usually have complications, e.g. bronchiectasis, deafness, enteroviral meningoencephalitis and neutropenia.

The treatment is lifelong immunoglobulin replacement every 6–8 weeks and maintenance of IgG to the level of IgG at 8 g/l. Infections should be treated, and physiotherapy should be given for bronchiectasis.

Referral should be made to a geneticist for all boys with XLA, as there will be risk for their offspring. All of their daughters will be carriers, but sons will be normal.

8. Answer: D

Neutropenia

Other causes are cyclic neutropenia, severe combined immune deficiency, chronic benign neutropenia and preleukaemia syndrome.

9. Answer: C

T-cell disorders

Severe combined immune deficiency, Omenn's syndrome, cartilage–hair hypoplasia, DiGeorge syndrome, and B-cell and T-cell combined disorders such as ataxia telangiectasia and Wiskott–Aldrich syndrome are all T-cell disorders. Patients are more prone to viral infection (e.g. respiratory syncytial virus, enterovirus and rotavirus), and mucocutaneous candidiasis, diarrhoea, and eczematous or erythrodermatous rashes should prompt suspicion of a T-cell disorder. Failure to thrive and poor weight gain are late signs of a T-cell defect. Opportunistic infection develops more commonly in an infant with poor weight, and can be the presenting symptom.

10. Answer: E

Complement deficiency

Deficiency of a complement protein, which is rare, is associated with autoimmune disease or increased susceptibility to infections. The complement components in the classical pathway are designated by a capital letter C and numbers 1–9. The two proteins participating in the alternative pathway are termed factors B and D. Proteolytically cleaved components of proteins are expressed by lower-case letters (e.g. C2a and C2b). Inactive components are designated with an 'i' (e.g. inactivated C3b is termed iC3b).

11. Answer: D (see answer to Question 7)

12. Answer: L

DiGeorge syndrome (DGS)

This can be inherited as AR, AD or X-linked. It is associated with dysmorphic features, cardiac problems, hypocalcaemia and cellular immune deficiency. Thymic hypoplasia or aplasia leading to defective T-cell function is one of the commonest immunological associations with DGS. There are complete and partial T-cell proliferative responses to mitogens. Partial DGS improves over time. Patients with complete DGS are rare and have no T-cell response to mitogens. These patients usually have very few detectable T cells in peripheral blood (1–2%) and generally require treatment. Blood transfusions should be used with caution in children with a significant T-cell defect because nonirradiated blood may prove fatal owing to a graft-versus-host response. Other manifestations that may be associated with DGS are growth retardation, and behavioural and psychiatric problems. Neurological abnormalities may include structural brain abnormalities and seizures, among others, and there may be genitourinary malformation. There may be an increased susceptibility to infections caused by organisms typically associated with T-cell dysfunction, which include systemic fungal infections, *Pneumocystis carinii* infection and disseminated viral infections.

13. Answer: F

Severe combined immune deficiency (SCID)

This is a life-threatening syndrome of recurrent infections, diarrhoea, dermatitis and failure to thrive caused by a number of molecular defects that lead to severe compromise in T-cell and B-cell functions. Patients usually present at about the age of 3 months with unusual severe recurrent infection or opportunistic infection.

SCID is divided into T-lymphocyte (T)-negative, B-lymphocyte (B)-positive and natural killer cell (NKC)-negative types. Most patients with SCID have an atrophic thymus with absent or severely reduced peripheral lymphoid tissues. Immunoglobulin and antibody production is severely affected even if there are enough B cells. Absence of cell surface proteins, including CD3, CD45 and major histocompatibility complex (MHC) class II prevents normal T-cell function and communication between T cells and other effector cells. Children with SCID will not show any physical abnormalities.

14. Answer: E

Leukocyte adhesion deficiency (LAD) type I

This is inherited in an autosomal recessive manner. It is not associated with defects in lymphocyte or antibody function. There is a failure to express the CD18 integrin, which serves as the receptor for C3b on myeloid and lymphoid cells. LAD is a rare disease. There is marked leukocytosis and localized bacterial infections that are difficult to detect until they have progressed to an extensive life-threatening level. The infections act similarly to those observed in neutropenic patients as a result of the inability of phagocytes to adhere to the endothelium and transmigrate into tissues. In LAD I, lymphocyte functions requiring LFA-1 (the CD2 pathway) are impaired. Delayed umbilical cord separation after the normal range (up to 3 weeks) is the classic presentation for LAD I.

15. Answer: I

Acute graft-versus-host disease (GVHD)

The presentation of acute GVHD involves a triad of dermatitis, hepatitis and gastroenteritis. Symptoms may occur alone or in different combinations. Other tissues that may be involved include mucous membranes, conjunctivae, exocrine glands, bronchial tree and urinary bladder. A maculopapular rash may be present, with onset occurring within 5–47 days after transplantation. Pruritis involving the palms and soles may precede the rash. The liver is the second most common organ involved. Elevated liver aminotransferases (transaminases) with cholestatic jaundice are common. Hepatic failure with encephalopathy is unusual. The distal bowel and colon are mostly affected, and patients experience profuse diarrhoea, intestinal bleeding, cramping abdominal pain and paralytic ileus.

Infectious Diseases and Microbiology

BOFs

1. The following are true about congenital infections except:

   A *Chlamydia trachomatis* in mothers can be treated with azithromycin.

   B Only HBe antibody-negative babies and mothers known to be HBsAg-positive should be immunized.

   C Mothers with genital HSV infections should be delivered by caesarean section.

   D Zidovudine should be given to all babies whose mother have AIDS or are HIV-positive.

   E Babies of mothers with active TB should receive isoniazid and BCG.

2. All of the following about neonatal bacterial infection and the best antibiotics are true except:

   A *Haemophilus influenzae*: cefotaxime

   B *Pseudomonas aeruginosa*: aziocillin and gentamicin

   C Group B streptococcus: ceftazidime and ampicillin, initially

   D Methicillin-resistant *Staphylococcus aureus*: vancomycin and teicoplanin

   E *Listeria monocytogenes*: ampicillin and gentamicin

3. The following descriptions of rashes and infections in children are all true except:

   A Hand, foot and mouth disease: vascular rashes

   B Fifth disease: maculopapular and reticular rashes

   C Glandular fever: maculopapular and punctate rashes

   D Measles: petechial rashes

   E Rubella: petechial rashes

4. The likely causes of pyrexia of unknown origin include the following except:

   A Lyme disease

   B Atrial myxoma

   C Thyrotoxicosis

   D Urinary tract infection

   E Shigellosis

5. The following organisms do not cause commonly acquired pneumonia in the age group of 3 months–5 years except:

A *Staphylococcus aureus*
B *Haemophilus influenzae*
C *Streptococcus pneumoniae*
D *Mycoplasma* spp.
E Group A streptococci

6. The following are false regarding *Escherichia coli* except:

A It is a Gram-negative motile bacillus.
B Differentiation between strains can be performed using various antigens on the organism.
C The enteropathogenic strain will cause watery diarrhoea by adherence and effacement.
D The enteroinvasive strain will cause bloody diarrhoea.
E The enterohaemorrhagic strain will invade the mucosa and cause non-bloody diarrhoea.

7. The following are true about varicella zoster except:

A It is a DNA virus.
B The infective period is 2 days before the eruption of rash and 5 days from the last eruption.
C Shingles can occur in children without a history of chickenpox.
D Aciclovir has no effect on the course of illness in immunocompromised patients.
E VZIG should be given to immuncompromised patients when there are any suspicions of contact with chickenpox patients.

8. The following are features of a gonococcal infection except:

A It is caused by a Gram-positive diplococcal bacterium.
B Neonatal ophthalmia appears within the first 5 days of life if the mother is infected with *Neisseria gonorrhoeae*.
C Systemic spread is uncommon.
D Chloramphenicol for the eyes is recommended for gonococcal ophthalmia neonatorum.
E Doxycyclin is the drug of choice for children above 12 years of age.

9. The following are criteria of *Haemophilus influenzae* and its complications except:

A It is a Gram-negative bacterium.
B There are six serotypes defined by polylipids on the capsule.
C Type B is the most virulent.
D Neonatal infection is caused by non-typable *H. influenzae*.
E Ceftriaxone is the drug of choice to eradicate the infection.

10. **The Hib vaccine is characterized by the following except:**

    A A polyribosylribitol phosphate (PRP) conjugate is the main vaccine.
    B A booster should be given to all children aged 4 years and above.
    C It has 95% effectiveness.
    D Asplenia and functional asplenia increase the risk of infection with Hib, so these patients should be targeted for vaccination and persuaded to have one.
    E Capsulated type b initially shows no response to the vaccine.

11. **The following regarding helminths and the most effective drugs used in treatment are true except:**

    A Piperazine: *Ascaris lumbricoides*
    B Thiabenzoate: *Strongyloides*
    C Praziquantel: schistosomiasis
    D Praziquantel: ocular cysticercosis
    E Diethylcarbamazine: *Toxocara* visceral larva migrans.

12. **The following are true about the hepatitis B virus except:**

    A It is an RNA virus.
    B It is a double-shelled particle with an outer lipoprotein envelope.
    C The core of the virus contains HBeAg and HBcAg.
    D Infectivity is high in patients with HBsAg and HBeAg.
    E Positive HBsAg, anti-HBc IgG, positive IgM, negative anti-HBs, positive HBeAg and negative anti-HBe are indications of a chronic hepatitis B infection.

13. **The following are true about human herpesviruses and the illnesses they cause except:**

    A HHV-6: exanthem roseola subitum
    B HHV-1: genital herpes
    C HHV-3: orolabial herpes
    D HHV-4: glandular fever
    E HHV-8: kaposi's sarcoma

14. **Infections with malarial organisms are characterized by all of the following except:**

    A 90% of patients infected with *falciparum* malaria can present within the first month of exposure.
    B Splenomegaly occurs in more than 90% of affected cases.
    C Cerebral malaria is commonly associated with *falciparum* malaria.
    D Hypoglycaemia is a common complication.
    E Oral chloroquine will be effective in *Plasmodium vivax, P. ovale*, and *P. malariae*.

15. The following are true about rotavirus except:

A It is an RNA virus.
B It is divided into seven serotypes and is the largest cause of infection in children.
C The incubation period is 6–12 hours.
D It does not infect the stomach or colon.
E Electron microscopy will identify rotavirus serotypes better than cultures.

16. The following are true regarding staphylococcal infections except:

A All staphylococci are coagulase-negative.
B Enterotoxins produced by *Staphylococcus aureus* will cause food poisoning and scalded skin syndrome.
C Food poisoning due to *S. aureus* enterotoxin will cause symptoms 30 minutes–6 hours after infection.
D Coagulase-negative staphylococci include *S. epidermidis* and methicillin-resistant *S. aureus*.
E Most *S. aureus* are β-lactamase producers.

EMQs

17–20. From the following scenarios, choose the appropriate investigation for possible causes of PUO from the list below:

17. A 6-year-old boy presents with a history of an intermittent fever for the last 4 weeks. This started as a sore throat with lymphadenopathy that has now subsided. The temperature can go up to 38.5°C every night. His CXR was reported as normal, and his full blood count showed atypical lymphocytes but no lymphoblasts. His spleen is 3 cm and not tender. His blood culture, blood film and viral serology for parvovirus are reported as normal.

18. A 13-year-old girl presents with a temperature and pains in her legs and had been unwell for 3 weeks. She has a fever almost every day. She was given oral co-amoxiclav for 5 days, which helped to stop the high temperature. Now she says that she is not walking. Her Hb is 11.2 g/dl and WCC 18.9 × 10⁹/l with neutrophilia. The ESR is 110 and CRP 95 mg/l. There is no joint swelling, lymphadenopathy, organomegaly, headache or meningeal signs. LP is reported as negative for meningitis.

19. A 17-month-old boy presents with a high temperature and has been unwell over the last 3 weeks. His parents have refused any vaccination since the age of 6 months. The current problem started as a sore throat, and on day 5 he developed maculopapular rashes. He developed bulbular conjunctivitis on day 7, but no organomegaly or lymphadenopathy. He looks miserable and is coughing. His CXR shows left lower lobe pneumonia, that was treated by IV ceftriaxone and oral azithromycin.

20. A 10-year-old girl presents with generalized lymphadenopathy, mainly in the inguinal region. She has been unwell over the last 6 weeks, with lethargy and a high temperature every 24–48 hours. She says that her body aches with the high temperature. Her lymph glands are mobile, and those at her groin are red and look inflamed. The FBC shows a low Hb of 8.7 g/dl, a WCC of 4.3×10^9/l and platelets of 125×10^9/l. Blood culture and serology for viruses and Lyme disease are all reported as negative. The CXR is reported normal, ESR is 15, and the CRP is fluctuating. She has had three courses of antibiotics without any benefit. Her family own a farm, and she says that she plays with her cats all the time. The dogs have been checked for any illnesses by the vet and have been reported as healthy.

Options
A Mantoux test
B ANA
C Double-strand DNA
D Bone scan
E Lower-limb X-ray
F Abdominal ultrasound
G IgM measles serology
H IgG serology for Lyme disease
I IgM for EBV
J Lymph node biopsy for cat scratch disease
K LP
L Rheumatoid factors
M ESR
N Echocardiography

21–24. Choose from the following scenarios the most likely investigation(s) to obtain the diagnosis of infections in children from the list below.

21. A 7-year-old presents with jaundice and abdominal pain and is not feeling well. He has not been abroad or in contact with anyone with a similar problem. His sclera is yellow, there is hepatomegaly and his urine is dark. A clinical diagnosis of hepatitis A is suggested.

22. A 5-month-old presents to A&E with a 2-day history of coryzal symptoms. He is wheezy and tachypnoeic. His chest is full of crackles, and bronchiolitis is the diagnosis. An NPA is done and sent to the laboratory.

23. A 7-month-old presents with a crusty, dark rash on the face. He is treated for 5 days with flucloxacillin. His rash does not improve, and initial swabs show no bacterial growth. The rash becomes vesicular in some parts of the face and on the neck.

24. A 2-year-old has refused to walk over the last 24 hours. He is miserable and looks febrile and septic. His left knee is swollen and red. Ultrasound shows fluid in his left knee, which is drained, and a sample is sent to the laboratory.

Options
A   Acid-fast bacilli film
B   Aspirated fluid culture
C   Blood culture
D   CRP
E   Human leukocyte antigen
F   Immunofluorescence antigen detection
G   ELISA
H   PCR
I   Electron microscopy for virus identification
J   ESR
K   Virus culture
L   Hepatitis A virus IgM

25–28. Choose the most appropriate antibiotic for the following infections from the list below:

25. A 3-year-old is brought to A&E with a swollen left eye. Orbital cellulitis is diagnosed.
26. A baby girl presents with a history of oral thrush for the last 3 weeks. She is treated with nystatin orally, but without improvement.
27. A 15-year-old girl presents with a history of vaginal discharge, and *Trichomonas* is isolated from the vaginal swab.
28. An 8-year-old girl presents with a history of a productive cough, weight loss and a mild temperature. The chest X-ray shows right upper lobe consolidation with hilar lymphadenopathy and a strongly positive Heaf test.

Options
A   IV flucloxacillin
B   IV ceftriaxone
C   Oral erythromycin
D   Oral cefixime
E   Oral penicillin
F   IV penicillin
G   Isoniazid
H   Oral tetracycline
I   Oral metronidazole
J   Oral ketoconazole
K   Rifampicin
L   Fusidic acid
M   Trimethoprim

29–32. The following scenarios concern tuberculosis. Choose the best management from the list below:

29. A 3-year-old is diagnosed with pulmonary and glandular tuberculosis.
30. A 15-year-old girl is diagnosed with tuberculous meningitis. Initially, she presented with a headache, photophobia and vomiting.
31. An infant is born to a mother with pulmonary tuberculosis.
32. A 3-year-old comes from the trace clinic with a Mantoux test of less than 7 mm, after having been vaccinated against tuberculosis at 7 days of age.
33. A 14-year-old girl just arrived from Pakistan with a history of pulmonary tuberculosis receives a 9-month course of isoniazid and rifampicin. She is still symptomatic and is coughing sputum with blood. The mycobacterium is resistant to both isoniazid and rifampicin.

Options
A Isoniazid for 3 months
B Isoniazid for 12 months
C Rifampicin for 12 months
D Give BCG if a tuberculin test is negative
E Isoniazid for 3 more months if a tuberculin test is positive
F Isoniazid for 6 months
G Rifampicin for 6 months
H Ethambutol for the first 2 months
I Steroids
J Pyrazinamide for the first 2 months

Answers for Infectious Diseases and Microbiology

1. Answer: B

Congenital infection

For HBsAg-positive mothers and HBe antibody-positive babies, only the babies should be immunized. For HBe antibody-negative babies and HBsAg-positive mothers, babies should be immunized and given HB immunoglobulin. In a confirmed or suspected HSV infection, aciclovir should be given to babies. There is no evidence that HCV is transmitted by breast milk. An infant with mother active TB status should receive isoniazid and rifampicin for 6 months. In toxoplasmosis, if the mother is acutely infected, she should receive spiromycin and serology should be done. If serology is confirmed on a newborn, pyrimethamine, sulfadiazine and folinic acid, alternating with spiromycin, should be given for a period of 3–6 months. If the mother is seronegative for chickenpox and there is a history of contact with chickenpox, she should receive varicella zoster immunoglobulin (VZIG). Termination is not indicated, and aciclovir can be given for acute infection. If babies are infected (7 days before and 7 days after delivery), VZIG should be given. Before or after that time, VZIG is not needed. In perinatally acquired infections with chickenpox, consider aciclovir.

2. Answer: C

Neonatal bacterial infection

Group B streptococci need penicillin and gentamicin initially, and, if there is still no response, vancomycin and teicoplanin. For group A, penicillin will be enough, and for group D, ampicillin and gentamicin should be given initially and then vancomycin and teicoplanin. For staphylococci, use flucloxacillin and gentamicin. For *Escherichia coli* and *Klebsiella*, cefotaxime will be enough.

3. Answer: D

Rashes in newborn babies

Vesicular rashes are associated with chickenpox, dermatitis herpetiformis, eczema herpeticum, HSV, impetigo, insect bites and molluscum contagiosum. Maculopapular and punctate rashes are associated with enterovirus infection, Kawasaki's disease, measles, pityriasis rosea, roseola infantum and scarlet fever. Petechial or purpuric rashes can be associated with ALL, ITP, Henoch–Schönlein purpura, bleeding disorders and congenital infections.

4. Answer: E

5. Answer: C

Acquired pneumonia

Other common causes of acquired pneumonia include *Bordetella pertussis* and mycobacteria.

Frequent causes of acquired pneumonia in the age group of 3 months–5 years are *Streptococcus pneumoniae* and respiratory viruses, and in later years *Mycoplasma pneumoniae, S. pneumoniae* and respiratory viruses. Between the ages of 1 and 3 months, acquired pneumonia is mainly due to viruses, *Chlamydia* and mycobacteria. In the group of neonates to 1 month, the responsible organisms are Group B streptococci, *Escherichia coli*, respiratory viruses and enteroviruses.

6. Answer: E

Escherichia coli

There are five strains of *E. coli* that are used for epidemiological studies, each of which will cause diarrhoea, but by different mechanisms of action. The enteroinvasive strain will cause bloody diarrhoea by adherence and invasion of mucosa, and is usually accompanied by fever. The enterotoxigenic strain will cause watery diarrhoea by adherence and will produce enterotoxin. The enterohaemorrhagic strain will cause non-bloody diarrhoea by increasing cytotoxin production, adherence and effacement. The enteroaggregative strain will cause chronic bloody diarrhoea by adherence and possible toxin production.

7. Answer: D

Varicella zoster

This can be transmitted via close contact, droplets and/or through soiled materials. Ninety percent of adults are seropositive to human herpesvirus 3 (varicella zoster virus, VZV). The incubation period is 14–17 days. The primary infection will cause chickenpox, with prodromal symptoms of mild fever and eruption of a vesicular rash, more so on the trunk. After that, the virus remains dormant in the dorsal root ganglia, and, if activated, will cause shingles. In early pregnancy, it may cause abortion. Varicella zoster immunoglobulin (VZIG) may be given to high-risk patients, and IV aciclovir can be given to acutely infected high-risk people and can reduce the period of infection. In neonates, aciclovir can be given for 14 days. The use of aspirin in children with chickenpox should be avoided, as this can lead to Reye's syndrome. It is a good idea to test for VZ antibodies in patients who are going to have chemotherapy or who are immuncompromised, and in pregnant women who are likely to come into contact with chickenpox and have no clear history of a VZ infection. A live, attenuated vaccine is available and can be given from the ages of 9 months to 12 years as one dose; this will give at least 6 years' immunity in immunocompetent children.

8. Answer: D

Gonococcal infection

This is one of the sexually transmitted diseases that is increasing among the adolescent age group and young mothers. It can be symptomatic in adolescence, but usually presents with discharges, orchitis or even pelvic inflammatory disease. It is usually accompanied by *Chlamydia*, and anyone having either of these should be counselled for HIV and syphilis testing. Treatment should be aggressive for neonates, with parenteral penicillin for 7 days and local chloramphenicol. In children under the age of 12 years (in which case it may be caused as a result of sexual abuse), ampicillin or penicillin should be given. In adolescents and children over 12 years, doxycyclin will cover both *Chlamydia* and *Neisseria gonorrhoeae*.

9. Answer: B

10. Answer: B

Haemophilus influenzae

There are six serotypes of polysaccharide on the bacterial capsule. There are other non-typable forms, which are responsible for neonatal infections and some infections in immunocompromised patients. Hib is responsible for 70% of meningitis and 10% of epiglotitis and cellulitus. Osteomyelitis and joint infections are less frequent. Third-generation cephalosporins are the most effective antibiotics, but sensitivity should always be determined when a culture is positive. A polymerase chain reaction can be performed if antibiotics are started or cultures are negative. The vaccination almost eradicates the infection if it is type b. There is a small group (<5%), who are not immune either because of poor technique or because the vaccine has not been updated. Other groups show low levels of antibodies and may require a booster. A new vaccine is available that will cover most serotypes.

11. Answer: D

Anti-helminths

Piperazine is used in the treatment of *Ascaris lumricoides*. Thiabenzoate is used also for *Toxocara* visceral larva migrans. Praziquantel is used in the treatment of neurocysticercosis – but not ocular cysticercosis or hydatid disease. Mebendazole is used in the treatment of threadworms and *Ascaris lumbricoides*. Albendazole is used in the treatment of *Strongyloides* and hydatid disease.

Corticosteroids can be used in acute infections with neurocysticercosis, *Toxocara* larva migrans, schistosomiasis and trichinosis. Surgery is used in hydatid disease and cysticercosis.

12. Answer: A

Hepatitis B

This is a DNA virus with a lipoprotein envelope and contains HBsAg. Carriers who are HBsAg-positive but have antibodies to the e antigen (anti-HBe-positive) are lower in their infectivity. Perinatal transmission from HBeAg-positive (anti-HBe-negative) mothers is approximately 80% if vaccine and immunoglobulin are not given. Transmission after the perinatal period is very low. If HBsAg, anti-HBc IgG, IgM and anti-HBe are positive and anti-HBs and HBeAg are negative, this indicates a hepatitis carrier with low infectivity. If HBsAg and HBeAg are positive and anti-Hbc IgG, IgM, anti-HBe and anti-Hbe are negative, this indicates a very early infection with a late incubation period. If HbsAg, anti-HBc IgG, IgM, HBeAg(+/−) and anti-HBe(+/−) are positive and anti-HBe is negative, this indicates acute hepatitis. If anti-HBc(+), anti-Hbs(+/−), anti-HBe(+/−), HBsAg, IgM and HBeAg are negative, this indicates immunity as a result of a previous infection. If HBsAg, anti-HBc IgG, IgM HbeAg and anti-HBe are negative and anti-HBs is positive, this indicates immunity because of immunization.

13. Answer: B

Herpesviruses

- HHV1 (herpes simplex virus type I, HSV-I) causes orolabial herpes, conjunctivitis, genital herpes, whitlows and meningoencephalitis.
- HHV-2 (herpes simplex virus type II, HSV-II) causes genital herpes, meningoencephalitis and orolabial herpes.
- HHV-3 (varicella zoster virus, VZV) causes chickenpox, encephalitis and shingles.
- HHV-4 (Epstein Barr virus, EBV) causes glandular fever, Burkitt's lymphoma, Hodgkin's lymphoma and nasopharyngeal carcinoma.
- HHV-5 (cytomegalovirus, CMV) causes glandular fever, congenital infections, retinitis, pneumonitis, enteritis, hepatitis and encephalitis in immunocompromised patients.
- HHV-6 and HHV-7 cause exanthem (roseola) subitum.
- HHV-8 causes Kaposi's sarcoma.

14. Answer: B

Malaria

The incubation period can extend from a few weeks to 5 years. Ten per-cent of *Plasmodium falciparum*-infected patients may present after 4 months. Splenomegaly is only present in less than 50% of infected patients, and hepatomegaly is less common. Hypotension, diarrhoea and septicaemia are other complications associated with a malarial infection. Renal failure, haemoglobulinuria and haemolytic anaemia are other complications more common with a *P. falciparum* infection. Nephrotic syndrome can complicate *P. malariae* and tropical splenomegaly with pancytopenia; hypergammaglobulin-aemia is related to recurrent exposure to *P. falciparum*. The treatment for *P. falciparum* includes admission until the parasites are <1% and oral quinine has been administered for 3 days, followed by Fansidar (pyrimethamine with sulfadoxine) as a single dose. If Fansidar is contraindicated in patients with a G6PD deficiency, mefloquine or tetracycline should be given (if the patient is aged above 12 years). In severe *P. falciparum* infection, intravenous quinine should be given every 8–12 hours until the parasite level is <5%.

15. Answer: C

Rotavirus

The incubation period is 2–4 days. It does not cause other systemic infections apart from diarrhoea and vomiting. It is possible to grow rotavirus in a tissue culture, but this is of no value. Electron microscopy is a diagnostic tool. Anti-gen detection in faeces is possible by ELISA, latex particle agglutination and radioimmunoassay. Genome detection directly from faeces is possible and are sensitive, specific and inexpensive. Antibodies have no value.

16. Answer: A

Staphylococci

Staphylococci are Gram-positive bacteria, with *S. aureus* producing a coagu-lase enzyme (coagulase-positive), while coagulase-negative staphylococci in-clude *S. epidermidis* and methicillin-resistant *S. aureus* (MRSA), which can cause nosocomial infections. Impetigo, paronychia, boils, wound infections, infected eczema and cellulitus are among the surface infections caused by staphylo-cocci infections. Deep infections such as periorbital cellulitus, scalded skin syndrome, pneumonia, septicaemia, osteomyelitis, urinary tract infections and meningitis are caused mainly by *S. aureus*.

17–20. Answers:

    17. A, B, C, I, L, M, N
    18. D
    19. G
    20. J

Pyrexia of unknown origin

The initial investigations for PUO should include FBC, thick blood film, repeated blood culture, EBV serology and saved serum for toxoplasmosis and CMV. More tests can be performed if the condition does not resolve; these include ESR, ANA, double-strand DNA, CXR and MSU, and LP should be considered.

Further testing will include a repeat blood culture, abdominal ultrasound, echocardiography, Igs, biopsy of any lesions or large lymph nodes, and a bone scan if there is any bone tenderness. White cell scans and a bone marrow biopsy should be left until after referral to the infectious disease team.

A study by Steel et al showed that, out of 100 children presenting with PUO, 22 had infectious causes, 6 autoimmune disorders and 2 malignancies, but that in the majority of cases no cause could be found.

21–24. Answers:

    21. K
    22. F, K
    23. F, K, L
    24. B, C, D, J

There are many non-specific tests for a suspected bacterial infection, including: full blood count, ESR, CRP, α-antitrypsin, cytokines, endotoxin, and CSF lactate, protein and glucose. Specific tests that will look specifically for the organisms that cause the infection include cultures for fluids, serology tests for viruses, DNA extraction looking for specific organisms, and histology from a biopsy.

25–28. Answers:

    25. A, F
    26. J
    27. H
    28. G, K

29–32. Answers:

29. F, G, H
30. B, C, H, I, J
31. A, D, E
32. A, D, E
33. R, H, J

Mycobacterium tuberculosis

Mycobacterium tuberculosis is a weakly Gram-positive bacillus that grows slowly in vitro and in vivo. It forms stable (fast) complexes with dyes that are resistant even to the presence of acid and alcohol and show red in colour when stained with Ziehl–Neelsen stain. *M. bovi* occurs in around 1.5% of cases if isolated. The incubation period is around 1–3 months. It is transmitted by small droplets from adults with open pulmonary tuberculosis. Congenital tuberculosis will present with non-specific symptoms, hepatosplenomegaly, fever, leukopenia and jaundice. It should be treated like extrapulmonary tuberculosis. The prognosis for most children with tuberculosis who are not immune-deficient is very good. In TB, the prognosis for meningitis if recognized early and treated early will be very good. Cavitation is very unusual in children, and if the organism is fully sensitive to treatment, an infected child will become non-infectious after 2 weeks of starting treatment.

Neonatology

BOFs

1. All of the following are causes of optic nerve atrophy in newborn babies except:

   A Hydrocephalus
   B Meningoencephalitis
   C Laurence–Moon–Biedl syndrome
   D Toxoplasmosis
   E Tay–Sachs disease

2. The following syndromes are recognized to be associated with cystic renal diseases except:

   A Tuberous sclerosis
   B Trisomy 18
   C Beckwith–Wiedemann syndrome
   D Down's syndrome
   E Zellweger's syndrome

3. The following are causes of macrocephaly in newborn babies except:

   A Subarachnoid haemorrhage
   B Post-haemorrhagic hydrocephalus
   C Vein of Galen aneurysm
   D Apert's syndrome
   E Cerebral malformations

4. The following are complications associated with RDS except:

   A Aspiration pneumonia
   B ASD
   C IVH
   D Subcutaneous emphysema
   E Acute renal failure

5. The X-ray findings in babies with transient tachypnoea of newborn are as follows except:

   A Hyperinflated lung fields
   B Increased vascular marking
   C Small pleural effusion
   D Hypergranulation
   E Perihilar opacities

6. **The following are common causes of seizures in the neonatal period except:**

   A Meningitis
   B Hypoxic ischaemic encephalopathy
   C Intracranial bleeding
   D Congenital abnormal brain
   E Hyperkalcaemia

7. **The following organisms do not usually cause bacterial meningitis in newborn babies except:**

   A Pneumococcus
   B *Escherichia coli*
   C *Listeria monocytogenes*
   D *Haemophilus*
   E Gram-negative bacilli

8. **The following are major clinical features associated with severe HIE except:**

   A Irritability
   B Coma
   C Prolonged seizures
   D Hypotonia
   E Absent suckling reflex

9. **Problems associated with SGA include all of the following except:**

   A Hypoglycaemia
   B Polycythaemia
   C Hyperthermia
   D Thrombocytopenia
   E Hypocalcaemia

10. **The following statements are true except:**

    A In newborn babies with persistent pulmonary hypertension, oxygenation is improved with nitric oxide inhalation.
    B Extracorporeal membranous oxygenation (ECMO) can be used in children with congenital diaphragmatic hernia to improve oxygenation.
    C High-frequency ventilation is associated with an increased incidence of pulmonary haemorrhage in premature babies.
    D In synchronized intermittent mandatory ventilation (SIMV), there is a significant increase in oxygenation.
    E Patient-triggered ventilation (PTV) is not superior to SIMV when weaning from conventional ventilation.

11. The following are the only causes of unconjugated hyperbilirubin-aemia except:

    A Hereditary spherocytosis
    B Galactosaemia
    C Polycythaemia
    D Congenital hypothyroidism
    E Cephalohaematoma

12. All of the following are true about bleeding disorders in newborn babies except:

    A Haematemesis or melena is most commonly due to blood swallowed by a baby.
    B Haemorrhages from the umbilical cord may be due to infection.
    C Vaginal bleeding is due to maternal oestrogen withdrawal.
    D Bruising on well babies is often due to infection.
    E Urinary tract system bleeding may be due to renal vein thrombosis.

EMQs

13–17. Chose from the following scenarios in newborn babies presenting with vomiting in the first week of life the most likely investigations from the list below:

    13. A day-old baby presents with frothy vomit. The pregnancy was normal, and the booked scan at 20 weeks was reported as normal. He is hungry and wants to feed, but the minute he is offered the bottle, he vomits and it is frothy. He has opened his bowels, with gas being seen in the stomach as well as a large bowel on abdominal X-ray.
    14. A premature baby born at 26 weeks is now 4 days old. He was ventilated for 19 hours and extubated on nasal CPAP with a PEEP of 6 and oxygen of 30 ml/l. He is on a feed of 1 ml per hour of breastmilk. His mother suffered from pregnancy induced hypertension and is now recovering. His oxygen requirement has increased in the last 3 hours, and he has become acidotic. His abdomen is distended, and he vomited bile.
    15. A week-old baby boy presents with continuous vomiting over the last 6 hours. He looks shocked and mottled. His sugar is 2.5 mmol/l and his blood pressure 40/60 mmHg. He is given fluids at 10 ml/kg of normal saline, and blood is taken. Benzylpenicillin and gentamicin are started as well. His urine shows increasing reducing substances. He is jaundiced, and his liver is about 3 cm below the costal margin. He is ventilated and kept nil-by-mouth over next 3 days. After extubation, he starts to feed again, but within 3 hours starts vomiting again, although his abdominal X-ray and ultrasound are reported as normal.

16. A 10-day-old baby boy presents with recurrent vomiting. He usually vomits 10–15 minutes after he has been given 5 oz of milk. He vomits all the milk and then wants to feed again. This happens three to four times per day. He is gaining weight now and has almost regained his birthweight of 3.760 kg. He is having up to 10 bottles per day. He is afebrile, and bowel sounds, blood gases and urine culture are all normal. There is no evidence of any clinical signs on systemic and general examinations.

17. A 3-week-old baby girl presents with repeated vomiting over the last 3 days. She looks dehydrated and is crying all the time. The vomit can sometimes be yellow, but she is also passing very jelly-like stools with blood mixed in. A stool culture shows no organisms after 2 days. She is on breast-milk. Her abdomen is distended at the time of presentation, with sluggish bowel sounds, and is tender on palpation.

Options
A Chest X-ray
B Abdominal X-ray and chest X-ray with large nasogastric tube
C Abdominal ultrasound
D Lateral cubitus abdominal X-ray
E Test feed
F Feeding history
G Septic screen
H GallPOT test
I Urine chromatography
J Urine amino acids
K Electrolytes
L Urinary 17-hydroxyprogesterone level
M Clotting screen
N Abdominal X-ray
O Barium swallow

18–20. The following scenarios concern respiratory distress syndrome. Choose from the list below the best way to manage these problems:

18. A 24-hour-old baby who was born at 26/40 was intubated at the age of 3 minutes, as there was no respiratory effort. There is a good heart rate, and two doses of Curosurf have been given. He is doing very well. In the last 30 minutes, he has started to look mottled and his CO_2 has risen to 7.9 kPa and the pH is 7.16, with a base excess of -4.2 and a PO_2 of 7.1. PEEP is 20/4, with an IT of 0.35 and a rate of 45. O_2 is 35%, with poor chest movement.

19. A 9-hour-old baby boy was born at 27/40 with good respiratory effort and good colour. He was transferred to a special care unit and within 30 minutes started grunting and was put on CPAP. Blood gas showed respiratory acidosis, with a CO_2 of 9.1. He was intubated, which was very difficult. Curosurf was given at the age of 2 hours. His ventilation set-up was 20/4, IT 0.4 and Rat 50. Oxygen dropped to 30% after Curosurf. A trial of UAC failed, but UVC was successful. A cranial ultrasound showed no evidence of IVH. By 9 hours, his oxygen requirement has gone up, and he is only saturated at 88% in 80%. The capillary blood gas shows a CO_2 of 8.8 and a pH 7.18, with a base excess of -6.3. His ETT is in place, as air entry is fine (at least on one side). He is receiving antibiotics, and his blood sugar is 6.1 mmol/l.

20. A 3-day-old baby was born at 25/40 of gestation. He was intubated aged 1 minute, given Curosurf and transferred to the NNU. He was given a second dose of Curosurf after 12 hours, which he tolerated well. He did very well on weaning conventional ventilation of PEEP 16/0.35 and a rate of 30. He is in air and about to be extubated next day. He is on day 2 of TPN, with fluid of 120 ml/kg/day via a long line. He has started to have desaturation, and his oxygen has gone up by 40%. There is no abnormal movement, air entry is equal and there is no pneumothorax. His electrolytes and CRP are within normal ranges. Arterial blood gas shows metabolic acidosis with a base excess of -11, CO_2 of 5.6 and pH 7.21. His Hb is 11.2 g/dl (at birth, it was 14.2 g/dl). Clotting is in the normal range, and platelets are 178.

Options
A   Check ETT
B   Abdominal X-ray
C   Echocardiography
D   Cranial ultrasound
E   Chest illumination
F   Chest X-ray
G   Check monitors
H   Repeat blood gas in 30 minutes
I   Check blood sugar
J   Re-intubate

21–25. From the following scenarios, choose the right diagnosis from the list below:

21. A newborn term baby started to have grunting at the age of 4 hours. The midwife found him to be tachypnoeic, mildly cyanotic and with a saturation of 85% in air. He was transferred to the neonatal unit and given 100%, but the saturation remained at only 90%. The air entry is reduced on one side and the blood gas shows respiratory acidosis. Blood pressure is 45/36 mmHg, with tachycardia.

22. A 2 week-old baby who was born at 26 weeks has been on a ventilator since he was born. Attempts to wean him and extubate him have failed twice. His chest X-ray shows an area of translucency throughout his lungs, with collapse as well. It has a snowstorm-like appearance. The chest is hyperinflated and with decreased chest wall movement.

23. A 7-day-old baby born at 25 weeks of gestation was treated for pneumothorax and is still on a ventilator. His blood pressure is not stable and he looks shocked and pale. The transverse diameter of the heart is reduced on chest X-ray.

24. A 4-day-old baby girl born at 24 weeks of gestation is on CMV with pressure 16/4 a rate of 35 and an IT of 1–1.5. The oxygen requirement has been rising and is now 40%. The baby looks pale, she is tachycardic and there is frequent desaturation. Blood-stained fluid appeared on suctioning the tube. The chest X-ray shows areas of consolidation and opacification.

25. A 10-hour-old baby presented with a history of apnoea and cyanosis as the midwife found him. He is crying and pink, and there appears to be no problem. His chest X-ray shows no abnormalities. A septic screen shows no evidence of infection, and he is on antibiotics. The blood gas is within the normal range, and echocardiography and cranial ultrasound show no abnormalities. He is observed on the NNU, and within 2 hours after sleep, he is found to be cyanotic, with the saturation falling to 66%. He is given facial oxygen and starts to cry and become pink.

Options

A Congenital lobar emphysema
B Cystic adenomatus malformation
C Pulmonary hypoplasia
D Pulmonary haemorrhage
E Air embolism
F Bilateral choanal atresia
G Pneumopericardium
H Pneumomediastinum
I Pneumothorax
J Pulmonary interstitial emphysema
K Chronic lung diseases
L RDS
M IVH
N Congenital heart diseases
O Congenital pneumonia
P Persistent pulmonary hypertension

26–30. **For the following scenarios, choose the right ways to manage these newborn babies from the list below:**

26. A 24-hour-old baby was checked and was due to be discharged home. He had apnoea and developed grunting. He was admitted to the unit and was found to be very acidotic and to have an abnormally shaped heart on X-ray. His liver is 3 cm, but there is no heart murmur. His lung fields are congested, with a right ventricular dominance on ECG.

27. A 3-week-old baby boy presents with tachypnoea, poor feeding and FTT. His mother says that every time he is fed, he cries, gets tired and is very irritable. He is tachycardic, but has a normal pulse and pulse pressure. His blood pressure is 60/44 mmHg, his liver is 4 cm below the costal margin, and a pansystolic murmur can be heard on the left intercostal space, radiating to the neck.

28. A 13-day-old baby girl was admitted from home, as her mother found her in a pool of vomit and not responding. The mother said that the baby's heart was very fast, and she is conscious and opening her eyes. By the time she arrived at hospital, she was alert and wanting to be fed. Her examination showed no abnormalities. A cardiac 12-lead ECG was done and showed a short PR interval and broad QRS with delta waves. She was admitted 2 days later with a similar episode, and SVT was terminated by IV adenosine.

29. A 9-week-old infant was admitted with a history of increasing cyanosis and not feeding. The heart rate was 190 bpm, with intercostal recession. The saturation in air was 88%. These problems have occurred every day over the last 3 days, mainly after the baby wakes up. The second heart sound is a single, ejection systolic murmur, heard best on the upper left sternal edge. The lung fields are oligaemic. The ECG shows right ventricular hypertrophy with right-axis deviation. The echocardiogram shows a right-side aortic arch, VSD, pulmonary stenosis and a reasonable pulmonary valve size.

30. A 4-hour-old baby was found to be cyanotic. He was taken to the neonatal unit, where his saturation was 70% in air. After being given 100% oxygen for a hyperoxic test, his saturation improved only to 88%. He is acidotic, with base excess of −15 and pH of 7.12. The femoral pulses are palpable, and only an ejection systolic murmur can be heard over the pericardium. He is working hard to breathe and has become more cyanotic.

Options
A Flecainide
B Propanolol
C Start IV prostaglandin infusion
D Verapamil
E Regular adenosine
F Start digoxin
G Give DC shock of 2 mols/kg
H Correct acidosis
I Furosemide (frusemide)
J Intubate and ventilate
K Referral to cardiology unit
L Surgical repair
M Atrial septostomy

Answers for Neonatology

1. Answer: D

Optic nerve atrophy in newborns

There are many causes of this subtle sign. Perinatal damage can occur without a cause being found. Compression by hydrocephalus and tumours such as craniopharyngiomas is a possible cause. Metabolic causes are rare, but should be looked for – these include osteopetrosis, Tay–Sachs disease and Batten's disease. Retinal damage can cause optic atrophy in association with Leber's amaurosis, retinitis pigmentosa, Laurence–Moon–Biedl syndrome and Zellweger's syndrome. Some can be inherited in an autosomal recessive manner. Optic nerve hypoplasia, where the optic disc is small, is very rare. It can be associated with other ocular abnormalities and may cause blindness, but normal vision can also be preserved in many patients. Microphthalmos, aniridia, absence of septum pellucidum, hydranencephaly, porencephaly and leukomalacia are often associated with an endocrine problem.

2. Answer: D

Syndromes with cystic renal diseases

An increasing number of syndromes are associated with renal cystic diseases. Trisomy 21 is not associated with an increase in the incidence of renal cystic diseases, although trisomies 13 and 18, Laurence–Moon–Biedl syndrome, Neil–Pettla syndrome, Jeune's syndrome, orofacial–digital syndrome and triploidy are. Medullary cystic diseases can also be seen in newborn babies, and can be autosomal dominant or recessive. They are characterized by hyposthenuria, anaemia and retinal changes, and a diagnosis can be confirmed by renal biopsy. Microcystic renal disease will be found with congenital nephrotic syndrome. The major cystic renal anomalies in a newborn are associated with polycystic kidney diseases. The autosomal recessive polycystic kidney diseases can develop from birth, with poor production of urine, and may lead to Potter's syndrome. The autosomal dominant type, which can be detected in babies, is usually more obvious in adult life. Large multicystic kidneys can be associated with renal dysplasia, and a prenatal diagnosis can be made. Most of the time, the condition is unilateral, and the kidney does not function.

3. Answer: A

Macrocephaly in the newborn

A large head in a newborn baby can have prenatal or postnatal causes. Prenatal causes can be familial, X-linked congenital hydrocephalus, Proteus syndrome (hemimegaloencephaly and hemihyperatrophy), cerebral malformations (Dandy Walker cyst, Arnold–Chiari malformation, aqueduct stenosis and arachnoid cyst), craniosynostosis as in Apert's syndrome, obstruction by tumours or vein of Galen aneurysm, and post-haemorrhagic and post-meningitic hydrocephalus.

4. Answer: B

Complications of RDS

The baby may be normal at birth, but over a few hours becomes tachypnoeic with increased respiratory effort and expiratory grunting. With small very premature babies, there is no delay until all of these symptoms appear. These babies are usually not breathing at birth and they need support straightaway, with Curasurf given after intubation. Pre-Curasurf chest X-ray changes are a ground-glass appearance, an ill-defined heart border and an air bronchogram. In severe cases, the lungs appear opaque. The blood gas will show low PaO_2, low pH, high CO_2, low bicarbonate and a base excess. Surfactant starts to be produced by 22 weeks of gestation, and surges at 33–35 weeks of gestation and at birth. Prenatal steroids will help to increase the production of surfactant in mothers who are delivering prematurely. If the baby deteriorates while on ventilator with RDS, first check whether there is chest movement. If the chest moves equally then increase the FiO_2 and wait – if there is no improvement then check for pneumothorax, lung infection, IVH, cardiac problems or sepsis.

If there is no chest movement then try to adjust the ETT – if there is no improvement then increase the PEEP. Listen again: if one side is better than the other then pull the tube back and check for pneumothorax or pneumonia. If there is no improvement, consider re-intubation.

5. Answer: D

Transient tachypnoea of the newborn (TTN)

This is relatively common and affects large preterm or term babies. It usually starts about 1 hour after birth, with a respiratory rate of 120/min, subcostal recession, grunting and cyanosis (which is not always present). The anterior-posterior diameter of the chest increases, and another added sign on chest X-ray is fluid in the transverse fissure. Early GBS infection may look similar, but the baby becomes unwell very quickly with GBS. Anomalous pulmonary venous drainage may also look like TTN. If the child does not improve and needs ventilator support, echocardiography should be done to exclude this. O_2 is often needed for 1–3 days. Antibiotic cover should be given if in doubt.

6. Answer: E

Seizures in the neonatal period

Other causes are hypoglycaemia, hypocalcaemia and rarely hyponatraemia. The following should also be considered: sepsis, maternal drug withdrawal, benign familial neonatal seizure, pyridoxine dependence, hypertension and inborn errors of metabolism. Seizures can be subtle, tonic, clonic and myoclonic. Neuroimaging should be performed in babies with focal seizures or with neurological deficit, developmental regression and uncontrolled seizures. EEG can also be done, but after a detailed history has been taken and after other biochemical abnormalities, different seizure types and recurrence of seizures have been ruled out, and not with the first seizure.

7. Answer: B

Bacterial meningitis in the newborn

The organisms that most commonly cause meningitis and septicaemia in newborn babies are group B streptococci. Meningitis is more common in the first month of life than at any other time. Shocked babies at birth or after birth should be treated as septic babies, and support should be offered straight away. Meningitis should be confirmed by LP as part of the septic screen of such babies. Others may present as pale, lethargic, drowsy and not interested in feedings. Babies with these types of infection should receive 7 days of IV antibiotics if there is no meningitis, but if there is meningitis then they should receive 2 weeks. All babies with meningitis should have their hearing checked and be followed up for a year. There is an increased risk of seizures and developmental problems.

8. Answer: A

Severe hypoxic ischaemic encephalopathy (HIE)

These babies also have no respiratory effort and need respiratory support. Babies with moderate HIE will be lethargic and then may have seizures, differential tone in the legs more than the arms and a poor suckling reflex; they rarely require ventilator support. Mild cases are usually irritable and hyperalert, and have normal tone. They feed satisfactorily but are weak; no ventilator support is required and there are no seizures. Babies with severe encephalopathy may die acutely, and if they survive, the risk of brain damage is high. EEG monitoring is beneficial to assess prognosis during the acute phase. The presence of a low-amplitude, discontinuous or unreactive trace indicates a poor prognosis. Burst suppression that is prolonged with no recovery in between carries prognostic significance. Neuroimaging in the first weeks after the events can be very helpful when there are extensive changes in grey as well as in basal ganglia. The MRI at 6 weeks of age is more helpful.

9. Answer: C

Small for gestational age (SGA)

For SGA, the baby's weight should be below the 10th centile for gestation. SGA is more commonly associated with mothers who are heavy smokers, suffer from chronic illnesses, have pregnancy-induced hypertension or placental insufficiency, are in a poor socioeconomic situation, or consume excess alcohol. SGA can be associated with chromosomal abnormalities, congenital infection, and toxins such as alcohol, phenytoin and warfarin. Other problems that may be associated with SGA are neutropenia, hypothermia, infection, congenital abnormality (Potter's syndrome), meconium aspiration, pulmonary haemorrhage, and high cortisol levels.

10. Answer: C

Newborn ventilation

PTV and SIMV are not superior for weaning babies from ventilator support. SIMV increases oxygenation as the baby synchronizes respiration with the ventilator. In PTV, all of the infant's respiratory effort that is greater than the trigger threshold is rewarded by a ventilator breath. ECMO can also be used in infants with severe lung infection, meconium aspiration and persistent pulmonary hypertension. In high-frequency oscillation, there is a suggestion that there may be an increase in the incidence of IVH and leukomalacia, but further studies are required to confirm this.

11. Answer: B

Unconjugated hyperbilirubinaemia

The causes of mixed jaundice can be hepatic or post-hepatic. Hepatic causes include any congenital infection causing hepatitis, cystic fibrosis, galactosaemia, α_1-antitrypsin deficiency and fructosaemia. Post-hepatic causes include congenital biliary atresia, choledochal cysts and bile plug syndrome. Unconjugated hyperbilirubinaemia can have pre-hepatic causes (ABO incompatibility, Rhesus isoimmunization, red cell enzyme defect, septicaemia, UTI and any bruises or trauma during delivery), hepatic causes (breast milk and congenital hypothyroidism) and post-hepatic causes (paralytic ileus and upper intestinal obstruction).

12. Answer: D

Bleeding disorders in the newborn

Bruises on babies are due to trauma, low platelets or a coagulation factor deficiency (especially of factors VIII and X). If the baby is well, it is very rare for infection to cause these kinds of problems. The haemorrhagic diseases of newborn babies can cause umbilical, GIT, urinary tract, scalp and cerebral bleeding.

13–17. Answers:

13. B (tracheo-oesophageal fistula)
14. N (NEC)
15. H, I, J (galactosaemia)
16. F (overfeeding)
17. K, L, N, O (intermittent volvulus)

18–20. Answers:

18. A, J
19. E, F
20. D
See also the answer to Question 4.

21–25. Answers:

21. I
22. J
23. G
24. D
25. F

26–30. Answers:

26. J, C, K (left outlet obstruction)
27. L, K (VSD with CHF)
28. A (WPW with SVT)
29. B, K (FOT)
30. J, H, C, K (TGA)

Management of the cyanotic newborn

In left outlet obstruction, babies usually present with life-threatening episodes where they are cyanotic and in heart failure. This is usually for the first 24 hours, up to 72 hours. When the duct closes, the baby becomes ill, and the peripheral pulses weaken and fail. There is usually a marked parasternal right ventricular heave, loud second heart sounds and a soft non-specific murmur. Treatment is supportive initially, with ventilation and by keeping the duct open or by atrial septostomy. Surgical correction can be performed, but the mortality is high.

Children who are critically ill following a duct-dependent heart lesion will need intervention, as the mortality rate is 90% in the first year of life. In the first few days, the duct needs to be kept open, and correction of acidosis and ventilatory support need to be commenced. Atrial septostomy should be performed until a full correction can be carried out. Discuss all of these cases with a cardiologist, as the problems arising will provide good practice, and any management will be guided by them.

Community Paediatrics

BOFs

1. **The following are features of ADHD except:**

   A Overactivity
   B Impaired concentration
   C Not listening to instructions
   D Daydreaming
   E Impulsiveness

2. **The following are approaches to treating children with ADHD except:**

   A Using methylphenidate
   B Training and support for parents
   C Special education provision is not required
   D Individual therapy can be achievable
   E Involvement of local health, educational and welfare agencies is required

3. **The following are characteristic features of dyslexic children except:**

   A Children will fail to read despite adequate intelligence.
   B Reading is usually significantly below the expected level.
   C Dyslexia mostly occurs during childhood.
   D Phonological memory is impaired.
   E Difficulty in abstracting letter sounds leads to a failure to develop phonic reading strategies.

4. **Language delay can be caused by all of the following except:**

   A Conductive hearing loss only
   B Multiple birth
   C Autism
   D Epilepsy
   E Oromotor dyspraxia

5. **Sexual abuse in boys can be suspected if the following injury is seen:**

   A Damage to the urethral meatus
   B Orchitis
   C Bruising or petechial haemorrhages on the penis
   D Incised wounds on the penis
   E Red, linear or circumferential marks on the penis

6. **The following are signs associated with genital abuse in girls except:**

   A Attenuation of the hymen
   B Irregular, thickened or rolled edges to the hymen
   C Fimbriated hymen
   D Sexually transmitted disease
   E Scars at posterior forchette

7. **What does the medical input for children requiring fostering and adoption include?**

   A Aiding the assessment process for fostering or adoption.
   B Empowering the child to take responsibility for his/her own health at the 21st birthday.
   C Aiding the assessment and planning process for the child.
   D Ensuring the coordination and continuity of healthcare for the child when moving to a new place.
   E Updating reports for the court hearing.

8. **The roles of a doctor when a child is referred for adoption include the following except:**

   A Assessment of family history
   B Attendance at the adoption panel
   C Educational and psychological assessment
   D Discussion of previous health issues with new parents
   E Liaision with other health professionals about the child's health

9. **In the community, Down's syndrome requires the following scheduled health checks except:**

   A Thyroid blood tests at ages 1 and 3 years
   B Echocardiography at 6 weeks of age
   C Full audiology review done only at age 3 years
   D Between the ages of 5 and 19 years, 2-yearly vision/orthoptic checks
   E Paediatric reviews on an annual basis after the age of 5 years.

10. **The following are causes of cerebral palsy except:**

    A Periventricular leukomalacia
    B Cortical dysplasia
    C Congenital CMV infection
    D Multiple pregnancy
    E Interventricular haemorrhage

11. **The following are causes of concomitant strabismus except:**

    A Refractive errors
    B Neurological impairment
    C Poor vision
    D Orbital trauma
    E Posterior fossa tumour

12. **The following are true regarding head injury in children except:**

    A After head injury, there may be frontal lobe damage leading to attention and concentration problems
    B After head injury, there may be temporal lobe damage leading to impaired new learning
    C Post-traumatic seizures are more common in children than adults
    D Post-traumatic headaches may last for years
    E Dystonia can follow head injury

13. **The following can be used to manage nocturnal enuresis in children except:**

    A Oxybutynin
    B Enuresis alarm
    C Imipramine
    D Desmopressin DDAVP
    E Carbamazepine

EMQs

14–18. From the following scenarios concerning language development in children, choose the correct age of the child from the list below.

    14. An infant can point to indicate need, shows intense attention in response to speech over a prolonged period, understands people's names, talks to toys and people with a few single words with meaning.

    15. A toddler can say 6–20 single words, repeats a few words, identifies two to four familiar objects and can make a single request. He is able to go upstairs using two hands.

    16. An infant pays attention to human faces, can vocalize two to three different syllables and starts making noises to get attention.

    17. A child uses three-word sentences with meaning, can select an item from a group of five familiar objects on verbal command, plays with blocks and makes a tower of six blocks.

18. A child plays and imitates other children in their verbal and activity. He understands actions and selects the appropriate picture if asked to do so, often uses personal pronouns correctly, and repeats words. He goes downstairs without holding onto rails.

Options
A 10 months
B 12 months
C 3–6 months
D 24 months
E 36 months
F 30 months
G 18 months
H 22 months
I 48 months
J 60 months
K 6 months
L 3 months

19–23. Match the following descriptions of gaits in cerebral palsy with the appropriate type of cerebral palsy from the list below:

19. The child walks with flexed hips and knees as if falling forward with occasional sclerosing. The weakness is more pronounced in the lower limbs than the upper limbs.
20. The child walks with a widely based gait and has a tendency to fall. The muscle tone is hypotonic and later may become spastic, and cerebular hypoplasia will be seen on an MRI scan.
21. The child walks normally but with many abnormal movements. As he grows older, he will be more rigid and have difficulty in walking. Usually, intelligence will be preserved.
22. The child limps and walks by bringing the affected lower limb forward in circumduction away, with the upper limb on the same side held in the flexion position at the wrist, and with the elbow and shoulder rotated inward.
23. The child is mentally retarded, with spasticity of all limbs – more so in the lower limbs. He walks with the frame only and drags the lower limbs. He has bulbar palsy, and the adductors of the lower limbs are very tense. The child suffers from hip dislocation, scoliosis and severe constipation.

Options
A Ataxic CP
B Hemiplegic CP
C Mixed CP
D Dyskinetic CP
E Diplegic CP
F Quadriplegic CP
G Neuropathic CP
H Neuromuscular CP

Answers for Community Paediatrics

1. Answer: D

2. Answer: C

Attention deficit hyperactivity disorder (ADHD)

This is a neurodevelopmental disorder with an incidence of up to 2% of the child population in some countries. Children with ADHD can be overactive, fidgety and disruptive, have impaired attention and lack of concentration, are easily distracted, never finish a task, do not listen to instructions, are impulsive, have a lack of social awareness, and find it very difficult to tolerate frustration. This has implications for the child's life, siblings and parents. There are three types of ADHD: overactivity and restlessness; inattentiveness and distractibility; or impulsiveness and social disinhibition. There are no specific causes, but certain factors can influence ADHD, such as diet, early childhood attachment problems, adverse family influences and overstimulation. There is a strong genetic link, and assessment should be done by a joint effort of schoolteachers, parents and a community paediatrician. Connor's score sheets can be completed by teachers and parents. Children who have been abused or who are developmentally delayed, ill-disciplined or overactive can be misdiagnosed with ADHD. It is important to rule out these other conditions. Treatment can be long and involve a multi-agency approach with several strategies. School, parents, psychologists and medication are all needed to help these children.

3. Answer: C

Dyslexia

This is defined as an inability to read despite adequate intelligence, conventional instruction and sociocultural opportunity. It is a lifelong condition. Children will perform poorly on tests of verbal short-term memory, and their difficulties with word finding or rapid naming may suggest that they have problems retrieving the information. Dyslexia is usually familial, and some brain structural abnormalities can be found on brain autopsy – e.g. cortical dysplasia on sylvian fissures or other fissures and histological abnormalities of the temporal lobe and the geniculate body, as all of these are concerned with memory. Treatment will involve informed training in phonological skills, as this has a benefit on reading and spelling, especially when combined with teaching of the letter–sound relationship.

4. Answer: A

Language development in children

Any hearing loss can cause language delay, as can a multiple birth, pervasive developmental problems, and functional brain damage such as head injury or epilepsy or a specific language or speech problem. Structural abnormalities in the mouth and cerebral palsy can also cause language delay. Familial causes can also lead to language delay. Maternal depression, stress and deprivation, behavioural problems, and a large family all can contribute to language delay. There is no point in assessing children below the age of 2 years. The delay can be in phonetics, grammar, semantics or pragmatics. Most of these problems will improve. Children with delayed expressive language – such as only eight words at the age of 2 years – will carry on having problems. Understanding language will continue regardless of whether or not the child has good expressive speech. If this is associated with other problems, it will usually last.

5. Answer: B

6. Answer: C

Child sexual abuse (CSA)

The suspicion of sexual abuse arises once a proper history has been taken and discussed with seniors. The injuries occurring in boys who are sexually abused can be present at the time or evidence may still be there. In acute cases, a complete forensic examination should be performed, with photographs. A torn fraenulum in forced retraction of the foreskin, burns or scalds and the criteria in Question 5 make sexual abuse more likely. Anal penetration is more common in boys, and a full examination should be performed when looking for evidence of sexual abuse.

In girls, the signs will include hymen laceration, erythema, oedema, laceration or bruising of the genitalia, dilated urethral opening, vaginal foreign bodies, labial fusion, a notch off the hymen, an enlarged hymenal opening, sexually transmitted diseases, other signs of physical or emotional neglect, or the child's demeanour during examination – all of which will make the case for sexual abuse more likely. Forensic examination with photographs and a detailed history taken by the child protection team will help. Fimbriated, sleeved or septate hymen are seen in the newborn. Torsion of the testis, hydroceles, testicular tumours and orchitis do not indicate sexual abuse in boys. Skin diseases (lichen sclerosis and atrophicus in girls), vulvitis due to threadworms, bubble baths, poor hygiene, or trauma, vulvovaginitis, haemangiomas, midline white streaks, urethral prolapse, urethral polyps, scarring implying previous trauma or surgery, straddle injuries, and inflicted injuries (female genital mutilation or sexual assault) can all be included in the differential diagnosis. If unsure, ask the expert.

7. Answer: B

8. Answer: D

Fostering and adoption

The work for adoption and fostering is usually done by collaboration between social services, voluntary agencies and doctors. The role of the paediatrician is to identify the current and future health needs of children, to provide input into the whole process, and to follow it up continually. His/her role is also to ensure the current medical knowledge and to empower the child to take responsibility at the appropriate age. The role of a doctor in the adoption process will also include providing a full medical report and functional assessment, a medical report for the adoption panel and providing liaison after adoption for possible new information. The interview with prospective adopters around the time of placement to discuss health issues is vital, and allows, when agreed, any medical information to be passed to the adopters. The medical advisor leading the service should ensure that mechanisms for monitoring and evaluating work, as well as maintenance of professional standards, are in place. This can be achieved through working with multiple agencies involved with the process, reviewing all decisions and obtaining full reports on a regular basis about each child who has been fostered or adopted.

9. Answer: C

Annual check for children with Down's syndrome

From birth to 6 weeks of age, there is a need to check thyroid function, growth, eyes and hearing and to perform echocardiography. From 6 to 10 months, growth and vision should be checked and a full audiology assessment should be performed. At the first birthday, the child needs TFT with antibodies, visual assessment, growth and orthoptic examination. At 18–30 months, they need growth, visual and orthoptic examinations, a full audiology assessment, and a dental check. At age 3–3$\frac{1}{2}$ years, they need TFT and growth and full audiology assessments. At age 3$\frac{1}{2}$–5 years, they need visual and audiology assessments. Between 5 and 19 years, they need an annual paediatric review with growth checks, hearing checks every 2 years, vision/orthoptic reviews every 2 years and TFT every 2 years. [This is adopted from the *RCHR Insert for Babies with Down's syndrome*, 2nd edn.]

10. Answer: D

Cerebral palsy

The causes of CP include maternal placental illness, rubella, toxoplasmosis, intrauterine infection, neonatal sepsis and cerebrovascular insult, and can be inherited or genetic. The commonest CP is diplegic, rather than hemiplegic, dyskinetic or quadriplegic. Ataxic CP is rare. Perinatal cerebrovascular diseases are responsible for causing diplegic CP in the majority of affected patients. Unilateral PVL or cerebrovascular disease are primarily responsible for hemiplegic CP in the majority of cases. Dyskinetic CP is usually due to asphyxia, but is also associated with mixed CP. Ataxic CP is due to cerebular hypoplasia, as in Joubert's syndrome. Quadriplegic CP is usually associated with HIE, congenital infections and prenatal cerebrovascular insult. Epilepsy is associated with 50% of diplegic and hemiplegic CP, and 80% of quadriplegic CP; it is uncommon in dyskinetic CP but common in ataxic CP. The IQ is normal in dyskinetic CP, 70–normal in diplegic and hemiplegic CP, <50 in quadriplegic CP, and 50–normal in ataxic CP. Often, vision is affected in diplegic, hemiplegic and quadriplegic CP, and hearing is affected in dyskinetic, diplegic and quadriplegic CP.

11. Answer: D

Strabismus

Concomitant strabismus is most common in children. The angle of deviation will remain the same wherever the eye moves. There are many unknown causes of strabismus, but it is important in any refractory error or neurological problem. Incomitant strabismus is usually caused by neurological or mechanical problems, such as VIth nerve palsy or orbital trauma. Half of the patients referred for orthoptistic assessment for strabismus are normal. The covered-eye test can be performed. GPs can be trained to do this – it is very easy. A light is shined into the eyes, where one looks for the pupillary reflex. If it is centred in both eyes, this is normal. In case one is temporally situated, cover it centrally. If the abnormality becomes central, the child has strabismus. If the child is not yet 10 years of age, there could be a latent squint or an underlying neurological problem, and a full neurological examination is required.

12. Answer: C

Head injury

Seizures are less common in children than adults following a head injury. The seizure can be of any type, but a full history should be taken, as some cases may relate to frontal or temporal lobe injury symptoms and not seizures. Post-traumatic headache may be due to migraine – but migraine, depression and stress follow a head injury. Spasticity is another problem that may follow a head injury, and children are often labelled as having cerebral palsy. Many drugs will relieve the spasticity (e.g. baclofen), but a high dose can be sedating. Dantrolene is less sedating. Botulinum toxin injection and intrathecal baclofen are in use for relieving spasticity. Rhizotomy is another way to manage spasticity. Family support and support at school is vital.

13. Answer: E

Management of nocturnal enuresis

Nocturnal enuresis can be due to a lack of stability in bladder function, a lack of arginine vasopressin release during sleep or an inability to wake from sleep in response to the sensation of a full bladder. Imipramine is not often used – although some paediatricians still employ it. A detailed history with a full assessment will help in planning management. Under the age of 5 years, trials of charts, rewards and fluid restriction are the first steps. Then medication and desmopressin are more effective in nocturnal enuresis. However, if the child has day-and-night wetting, oxybutynin can help. Alarms are effective and can be tried before medication after the age of 5 years.

14–18. Answers:

14. B
15. G
16. C
17. D
18. F

19–23. Answers:

19. E
20. A
21. D
22. B
23. F

See answer to Question 10.

Inborn Errors of Metabolism

BOFs

1. Regarding inborn errors of metabolism (IEM) in children, the following are true except:

   A Most metabolic defects are recessively inherited.
   B At least 1–2% of the population have a pathogenic metabolic disorder, most of which are of little clinical importance in childhood.
   C Almost all of the IEMs are rare – many extremely so.
   D Most present in the first year of life.
   E In a child with a normal routine newborn screening result, the possibility of an IEM is almost excluded.

2. The common reasons for referral to metabolic clinics in childhood are the following except:

   A Lactic acidosis
   B Hyperlipidaemia
   C Rickets
   D Hypoglycaemia
   E Abnormal results from newborn screening

3. The following are false regarding investigating amino acid metabolism except:

   A Phenylketonuria is the only common IEM diagnosed by routine newborn blood screening tests.
   B The term 'aminoaciduria' indicates the presence of amino acids in the urine.
   C Generalized aminoaciduria usually indicates the presence of an IEM of amino acids.
   D In argininosuccinic aciduria and non-ketotic hyperglycaemia, the blood levels of argininosuccinic acid and glycine, respectively, are markedly elevated.
   E Adult rates of renal amino acid reabsorption are reached by 3–6 months of age.

4. The following are features of untreated phenylketonuria except:

   A Microcephaly
   B Abnormal EEG
   C Glaucoma
   D Eczematous skin
   E Mousy, musty odour

5. The following are features of phenylketonuria except:

A There are white matter changes on the brain MRI in untreated older children.
B Treatment started at 1 year of age improves the IQ significantly.
C Treatment (diet) is recommended lifelong.
D Treated patients may develop learning and behavioural problems if the diet is relaxed or stopped, which can reverse if the diet can be successfully reintroduced.
E In treated patients, phenylalanine should be kept below 600 μmol/l at all times.

6. The following are true regarding tyrosinaemia except:

A Neonatal hypertyrosinaemia disappears by 1 week of age.
B Neonatal hypertyrosinaemia is more common in preterm than term newborns.
C It causes liver cirrhosis.
D It causes generalized aminoaciduria.
E Hepatic carcinoma may be a complication in older patients.

7. The following are false regarding investigations in tyrosinaemia except:

A Liver and kidney function tests are normal, and the prothrombin time is not markedly prolonged.
B Detection of succinylacetone in fresh-frozen urine samples is diagnostic.
C Elevated blood tyrosine or methionine is diagnostic in a neonate with evidence of liver damage.
D Serum α-fetoprotein is low.
E Prenatal diagnosis is not yet available.

8. Tyrosyluria may be seen in:

A Cystic fibrosis
B Thyrotoxicosis
C Liver disease
D Normal people
E All of the above

9. The following are causes of hyperammonaemia except:

A Carbamoyl phosphate synthetase deficiency
B Cystathionine synthase deficiency
C Ornithine transcarbamoylase deficiency
D N-acetylglutamate synthetase deficiency
E Transient neonatal hyperammonaemia

10. The following are features of cystathionine synthase deficiency except:

A There is skin telangiectasia.
B About half of cases respond completely to pyridoxine therapy.
C Infants usually appear normal.
D Dislocation of the lens usually results in myopia.
E There is hepatomegaly with abnormal liver function tests.

11. Causes of hyperammonaemia include the following except:

A Methylmalonic aciduria
B Reye's syndrome
C Ketotic hypoglycaemia
D Valproic acid toxicity
E Ureterostomy

12. The following are true regarding the diagnosis of homocystinuria except:

A There is a high homocystine level in the plasma.
B The urine nitroprusside test is positive.
C Diagnosis is confirmed by urine chromatography.
D Plasma methionine is elevated.
E A neonatal blood-screening test is available.

13. The following are true regarding albinism except:

A The oculocutaneous form is due to a lack of tyrosinase enzyme activity, and it is an autosomal recessive disorder.
B The ocular albinism is an X-linked disorder.
C Patients with the oculocutaneous form have red pupillary reflexes.
D It has an incidence of about 2 per 1000.
E In the oculocutaneous form, there is a greatly increased risk of skin neoplasia.

14. The following treatment is not routinely needed in tyrosinaemia:

A Low-tyrosine diet
B Low-phenylalanine diet
C Vitamin D
D Vitamin K
E Vitamin A

EMQs

15–20. Match each of the following IEM with its treatment below:

15. Methylmalonic acidaemia
16. Hyperammonaemia
17. Maple syrup urine disease
18. Homocystinuria
19. Propionic acidaemia
20. Albinism

Options

A Sodium benzoate
B Tinted glasses
C Haemodialysis
D Folic acid
E Biotin
F Strict special diet
G Lactulose
H Massive doses of vitamin B_{12}
I Pyridoxine
J Thiamine
K Sunscreen preparations

21–26. Match each of the following clinical presentations with the most likely diagnosis below:

21. X-linked, cataract, buphthalmos, marked hypotonia, frontal bossing, cryptorchidism and severe failure to thrive. It is also associated with self-mutilation. The level of uric acid will be very high.
22. Progressive hypotonia, weakness, hyporeflexia, glossomegaly, massive cardiomyopathy, normal cerebral development and a huge QRS complex on ECG. There is hypoglycaemia that needs more than 15% dextrose infusion.
23. Intermittent photodermatitis, ataxia, psychiatric changes and mental deterioration.
24. Sudden infant death syndrome, recurrent hypoketotic hypoglycaemia, hepatic dysfunction and cardiomyopathy.
25. Generalized aminoaciduria, phosphaturia, glucosuria and failure to thrive.
26. Hepatosplenomegaly, progressive liver dysfunction, hypoglycaemia, anaemia, Fanconi's syndrome, cataracts and a positive clinitest.

Options
A Hartnup's disease
B Tay–Sachs disease
C Hurler's syndrome
D McArdle's syndrome (GSD type V)
E Pompe's disease (GSD type II)
F Tyrosinaemia
G Lowe's syndrome
H Medium-chain acyl-CoA dehydrogenase deficiency (MCAD)
I Galactosaemia
J Porphyria
K Fanconi's syndrome
L Lesch–Nyhan syndrome

27–29. For the following scenarios regarding epilepsy associated with metabolic disorders, choose the most appropriate investigations from the list below:

27. A 2-week-old baby presents with a history of altered consciousness, hypertonia and opisthotonos with seizures. Blood amino acid chromatography shows an increase in branched amino acids, leucine, isoleucine and valine.

28. A 4-day-old baby presents with hypothermia, is acidotic and dehydrated, exhibits loss of consciousness and starts to have generalized tonic clonic seizures. The EEG shows burst suppression. There is a characteristic odour of sweaty feet. There is ketonuria. There is a suspected diagnosis of iso-valeric acidaemia.

29. A 2-week-old baby presents with vomiting, anorexia, som-nolence and convulsions followed by coma. There is no acidosis or ketosis. The blood sugar is normal, and there is no organomegaly.

Options
A Serum lactate
B Serum ammonia
C Blood gas
D FBC
E Bone marrow aspirate
F Blood chromatography
G Pyruvate
H Transferrin isoelectrophoresis
I Urinary amino acids
J Urinary organic acids
K Uric acid level
L Urine odour
M Very long-chain fatty acids
N Free and esterfied carnitine

Answers for Inborn Errors of Metabolism

1. Answer: E

Metabolic disorders

Most metabolic defects are recessively inherited. At least 1–2% of individuals have a pathogenic metabolic disorder, most of which (e.g. hyperuricaemia and hyperlipidaemia) are of little clinical importance in childhood. Almost all of these conditions are rare (1 : 100 000–1 : 250 000); many are extremely rare (10^{-6}–10^{-7}). However, if there are 1000 diseases each occurring only one in a million, 1 : 1000 people will have one of them, and for *each* of these conditions, 1 : 500 is a carrier! They can disrupt the function of any organ and may present at any age to specialists in any clinical discipline. Routine newborn screening screens for an extremely limited number of diseases, and in no way does it exclude the possibility of an IEM.

2. Answer: B

Reasons for referral of suspected metabolic diseases

- Lactic acidosis
- Metabolic bone disease (vitamin D-resistant rickets)
- Abnormal results from newborn screens (phenylketonuria, MCAD)
- Polyuria (diabetes)
- Failure to thrive with visceromegaly (Gaucher's disease, etc.)
- Dysmorphic features with other organ involvement (mucopolysaccharidoses, etc.)
- Porphyria
- Neurological disorders with seizures in the first year of life
- Previously affected child
- Failure to thrive, with consanguinity

3. Answer: E

Amino acids

The term 'aminoaciduria' indicates that the urinary amino acids are greater than normal. Generalized aminoaciduria is more likely to be due to a renal tubular defect.

In some conditions, such as argininosuccinic aciduria and non-ketotic hyperglycaemia, the amino acids are excreted readily in the urine, and blood levels may be only mildly abnormal, although in both of these conditions the level is markedly increased in the cerebrospinal fluid.

The quantity of amino acids in the urine can vary over 10-fold in normal people and depends greatly upon age and nutrition. The levels are higher in infants, but the range is so wide that normal values are hard to establish. Normally, renal tubular reabsorption is nearly 100%, notable exceptions being histidine and glycine. In early infancy, many amino acids may be reabsorbed poorly, adult rates being reached by 3–6 months.

4. Answer: C

5. Answer: B

Phenylketonuria (PKU)

With rare exceptions, PKU, when untreated, causes progressive brain damage, with a loss of 40–60 points in the IQ by 1 year of age. By 1 year of age, microcephaly, eczematous or oily skin, hypertonicity, convulsions, dysphasia, hyperactivity with purposeless movements, and an abnormal EEG are usual. In early infancy, vomiting may mimic pyloric stenosis. The skin and hair are often fair, with blue eyes. Psychotic behaviour with hyperactivity, destructiveness, self-injury, impulsiveness and uncontrolled behaviour are noted. The general physical development is usually good.

Patients with PKU who are treated early generally have an intelligence within normal range. Hyperactivity and a lower IQ than a first-degree relative have been noticed in many patients with PKU. The frequency of abnormalities associated with EEG and MRI increases with age. Demyelination is almost universal in older patients affected with both classical PKU or HPA type II.

Plasma phenylalanine is elevated, and phenylalanine and its metabolites appear in the urine. Phenylacetic acid accounts for the subtle mousy, musty odour of these patients.

Many older children develop learning and behavioural problems if the diet is relaxed or stopped. These can reverse if the diet can be successfully reintroduced, but compliance may be extremely hard to maintain.

The level of phenylalanine at which brain damage can occur is not known. Treatment is started if the blood level exceeds 400–700 μmol/l. Elemental medical foods from which phenylalanine has been totally or partially removed are mixed with ordinary infant formula or cows' milk or combined with a breastfeeding regime so that the total intake of phenylalanine is reduced sufficiently to maintain the blood level at 150–600 μmol/l. Weaning with low-protein foods starts at the normal time, but the special formula usually remains essential. After 2–3 years, phenylalanine-free products remain the main source of protein and calories.

Treatment should start as soon as possible: if it is started in 2–3 weeks, the prognosis is excellent. If treatment is delayed by several weeks, the outcome is more variable. Patients treated after 6 months show some improvement in IQ, but they are likely to be brain-damaged. Older patients usually show little change in IQ. The diet should be continued as long as practical (lifelong if possible), with blood levels being monitored.

6. Answer: A

Tyrosinaemia

In about 5% of premature babies and some term newborns, gross tyrosinaemia and tyrosyluria with secondary hyperphenylalaninaemia may occur and last as long as 3 months. This is due to immaturity of liver enzymes, high protein intake, or possibly suboptimal vitamin C intake by the mother and infant.

Hepatocellular damage leading to cirrhosis and liver failure and renal tubular damage resulting in Fanconi's syndrome (with generalized aminoaciduria) are the hallmarks of hereditary tyrosinaemia. Failure to thrive, rickets, thrombocytopenia and a profound clotting disorder (which may resist therapy with parenteral vitamin K) are frequent. Hypertrophic cardiomyopathy may occur. There is a severe form with rapid deterioration and death in the first weeks of life and milder cases that may survive until adult life; both may occur in the same family. In older cases, hepatic carcinoma is very common.

7. Answer: B

Tyrosinaemia

Standard liver and kidney function tests are abnormal, and the prothrombin time is markedly prolonged. Plasma tyrosine and methionine are usually, but not invariably, elevated. Serum α-fetoprotein is very high, there is generalized aminoaciduria and tyrosyluria and δ-aminolaevulinic acid excretion is usually increased. Blood tyrosine or methionine may be elevated by hepatocellular damage due to other causes such as galactosaemia or any neonatal hepatitis. Detection of succinylacetone by gas chromatography in fresh-frozen samples of urine is diagnostic, since it is not excreted in other disorders. Confirmation by enzyme assay in cultured fibroblasts is feasible, but false normals have been reported. Prenatal diagnosis by enzyme assay or finding succinylacetone in the amniotic fluid is possible.

8. Answer: E

Tyrosyluria

Several diseases cause high plasma levels of tyrosine (tyrosinaemia) and excretion of tyrosine metabolites in the urine (tyrosyluria). These compounds reduce Benedict's solution and give a positive reducing-substances test.

Tyrosyluria occurs in scurvy, since step five in its metabolism is vitamin C-dependent. It is also reported in rheumatoid arthritis, liver disease, thyrotoxicosis and megaloblastic anaemia, and occasionally in normal people (where the cause is less well established). In malabsorption, such as cystic fibrosis, gut tyrosine is degraded by bacteria and tyrosyluria often occurs.

9. Answer: B

Hyperammonaemia

Cystathionine synthase deficiency causes homocystinuria. The other enzymes are enzymes of the urea cycle and their deficiency causes hyperammonaemia. Hyperammonaemia is also sometimes seen in infants receiving intravenous alimentation, mostly preterm babies. It may cause progressive neurological damage. Ammonia levels may be as high as 5 mmol/l. Liver function tests and amino acid studies may be normal. If the condition is treated early and vigorously, the babies rapidly improve and the prognosis is excellent. In infants who recover, the protein tolerance becomes normal, and liver enzyme assays show no abnormality. The cause is unknown.

10. Answer: E

Cystathionine synthase deficiency

Homocystinuria can be caused by defects either in cystathionine synthase or in the methionine recycling pathway. Different mutations of cystathionine synthase result in varying response to pyridoxine both in vivo and in vitro, but about half of such cases respond completely to pyridoxine therapy due to its effect in stabilizing the mutant enzyme.

Infants usually appear normal, but later osteopenia with kyphoscoliosis, pectus excavatum or carinatum, genu valgum and pes cavus are common. The appearance may resemble Marfan's syndrome with arachnodactyly and long limbs, but the hypermobility of the joints is not marked, with some patients showing few physical abnormalities. Dislocation (usually downward) of the lens develops, usually resulting in myopia and often in optic atrophy, glaucoma, cataract and retinal detachment. Commonly, the hair is fair and easily broken. The skin tends to become coarsened, with telangiectasia and acne. Hepatomegaly is caused by fatty infiltration; standard liver function tests are usually normal. About 50% of these patients are developmentally delayed, and those with normal intelligence often have psychiatric problems.

11. Answer: C

Causes of hyperammonaemia

The causes of secondary hyperammonaemia (not due to a urea cycle defect) include the following: liver disease, Reye's syndrome, lactic acidosis, ketotic hyperglycinaemia, methylmalonic aciduria, propionic aciduria, 3-ketothiolase deficiency, 3-hydroxy-3-methylglutaric aciduria, familial lysinuric protein intolerance, periodic lysinaemia with hyperammonaemia, neonatal glutaric aciduria type II, defects of fatty acid oxidation, valproic acid toxicity, ureterostomy, shock and after surgery.

12. Answer: A

Homocystinuria

The urine nitroprusside test is positive unless the urine is very dilute; confirmation is by chromatography of the urine. Homocystine is barely detectable in normal plasma, and even in these patients is only present in small amounts since it is rapidly cleared by the kidneys. Plasma methionine is elevated in cystathionine synthase deficiency, but it is normal or low in methionine resynthetic defects. A neonatal blood-screening test is available for hypermethioninaemia, but false-positive results can occur. Urinary methionine may be elevated, but care must be taken to distinguish D-methionine, which is contained in several infant formulae and is absorbed from the gut and excreted unchanged in the urine. The urine test usually becomes positive within a few days of birth, but may be delayed for up to 2 weeks. Carriers are best diagnosed by enzyme assay of cultured fibroblasts.

13. Answer: D

Albinism

The incidence of albinism is around 1 : 10–20 000. It is a common disorder. In oculocutaneous albinism, tyrosinase has no activity or some residual activity. The most severe albinism occurs in tyrosinase-negative patients, in whom the absence of pigment is complete and permanent. These patients have very pale hair and skin. They have no pigmented naevi or freckles, and there is a greatly increased risk of skin neoplasia. The iris is always blue or grey, there is marked nystagmus and photophobia, and most patients are legally blind. Lack of retinal pigment produces a red pupillary reflex.

In ocular albinism, the depigmentation is confined to the eyes: four variants are recognized, all of which are X-linked disorders.

14. Answer: E

Treatment of tyrosinaemia

Treatment of tyrosinaemia consists of a low-phenylalanine and low-tyrosine diet (300–500 mg/day), which may produce considerable improvement in clinical, biochemical and histological findings. Additional treatment for Fanconi's syndrome (e.g. 1,25-dihydroxyvitamin-D_3 or alkali) and for hepatocellular damage (e.g. vitamin K or dietary restriction of protein) may be required. A competitive inhibitor of pHPPA hydroxylase, known as NTBC, is extremely effective in reversing even severe liver damage and in reducing the level of succinylacetone to normal, but if liver damage is advanced then liver transplantation is indicated and should be performed as early as possible to prevent hepatic carcinoma. After transplantation, patients still excrete succinylacetone but appear to escape toxic damage to the transplanted liver. It is not known whether the drug can permanently prevent cancer.

15–20. Answers:

15. H
16. A, C, G
17. C, F, J
18. D, I
19. E
20. B, K

21–26. Answers:

21. G
22. E
23. A
24. H
25. K
26. I

27–29. Answers:

27. **I:** Maple syrup urine disease usually presents with neurological distress without acidosis. The immediate treatment will improve the outcome. Leukodystrophy may show on MRI due to spongiosis.
28. **A, B, C, D:** Isovaleric acidaemia usually presents with neurological distress and ketoacidosis. The prognosis depends on the time of diagnosis. Enzymatic deficiency can be recognized in similar conditions, such as methylmalonic acidaemia, propionic acidaemia, β-oxidation defects and glutaric aciduria type II, all of which can be diagnosed by performing chromatography of amino acids and urine organic and amino acids. A liver biopsy looking for the enzyme deficiency can be also helpful.
29. **B, C:** Urea cycle defects will present at early stages as soon as feeding is started. If it is not recognized and treated, patients will die within the first 48 hours. Urgent dialysis is the treatment of choice.

Respiratory Medicine

BOFs

1. The following are true about surfactant except:

   A It is produced by alveolar type I epithelial cells.
   B It can be detected at the alveolar surface by 30 weeks of gestation.
   C Its synthesis is enhanced by cyclic adenosine monophosphate (cAMP).
   D Its synthesis is inhibited by insulin.
   E Storage can be identified in type II epithelial cells at 24 weeks of gestation.

2. Common viruses responsible for otitis media include all of the following except:

   A Respiratory syncytial virus
   B Parainfluenza virus
   C Adenovirus
   D Influenza virus
   E Rhinoviruses

3. The most appropriate investigation in infants with bronchiolitis is:

   A Chest X-ray
   B Arterial blood gas
   C Blood culture
   D Nasopharyngeal aspirate
   E None of the above

4. The following are common viral causes of pneumonia in children except:

   A Respiratory syncytial virus
   B Adenovirus
   C Influenza B
   D Parainfluenza
   E Coxsackie

5. Uncommon bacterial causes of pneumonia in infants and young children include all of the following except:

   A *Haemophilus influenzae* type b
   B *Streptococcus pneumoniae*
   C *Staphylococcus aureus*
   D Group streptococci
   E *Pseudomonas aeruginosa*

6. A 10-year-old boy presents for the first time with difficulty in breathing and shortness of breath. He is not a known asthmatic, but there is a family history of atopy. There are expiratory wheezes and a few crackles on listening to his chest. He responds to salbutamol inhalers of 10 puffs that are needed every 2 hours. He is admitted and given prednisolone at 40 mg once a day for 3 days. All of the following regarding management are false when this changed except:

A Use salbutamol inhalers when needed
B Inhaled steroids every day
C Regular salbutamol inhaler
D Lung function test
E Regular asthma clinic follow-up

7. A 7-year-old girl is a known asthmatic and is on regular budesonide 200 μg/twice a day via a spacer and a salbutamol inhaler, of which she uses two puffs twice a day via a spacer. She cannot sleep at night because of coughing and is tired during the day. The management plan should involve the following except:

A Increase budesonide to 400 μg/twice a day.
B Check her techniques using the inhalers.
C Add leukotriene receptor antagonist at 5 mg once a day.
D Long-acting β-antagonist once every day
E Regular asthma clinic follow-up

8. An 11-year-old boy is a keen footballer but has found it very difficult to finish games. He is a known asthmatic and is on regular Flixotide (fluticasone propionate) at 250 μg twice a day via an Accuhaler and also uses salbutamol at 4–6 puffs via an Accuhaler before and halfway through the match. His technique is very good, and his follow-up with the asthma clinic is regular. What is the most appropriate action from the following?

A Refer to an asthma specialist
B Change the inhaled steroids
C Check lung function test
D Arrange for a bronchoscopy
E Add singulair

9. A 5-year-old girl presents to A&E with a history of difficulty in breathing. She is sitting, not talking, and looks very anxious. Her saturation in 5 l of oxygen via a facemask is 90%. She is using her accessory muscles and is a known asthmatic. She was playing outside when her mother found her crying and noticed that her breathing was very shallow. She gave her 10 puffs of salbutamol via a spacer and brought her to hospital. What are the plans of action for this patient?

A Give back to back of 5 mg nebulized salbutamol
B Intravenous hydrocortisone
C Consider salbutamol infusion
D Arterial blood gas
E All of the above

10. Involvement of the lungs in cystic fibrosis can be any the following except:

A Pneumothorax
B Bronchiectasis
C Bronchitis
D Alveolitis
E Haemoptysis

11. Complications associated with cystic fibrosis include the following except:

A Nasal polyps
B Infertility
C Portal hypertension
D Cholethiasis
E None of the above

EMQs

12–16. From the following scenarios, choose the most appropriate diagnosis from the list below:

12. A 2-year-old boy presents with difficulty in breathing, a barking cough, and inspiratory and expiratory stridor. He is afebrile, with a saturation of 93% in air.

13. A 3-month-old baby girl presents with difficulty in breathing, with a respiratory rate of 50/min, tachycardia and intercostal recession, and is afebrile. She has been snuffly for the last 2 days. Examination reveals inspiratory stridor. There are no other abnormalities apart from a birthmark on her scalp.

14. A 6-week-old baby boy presents with funny noisy breathing. It is worse when he is asleep or has been fed. There is mild recession and no dysmorphic features or birthmarks.

15. A 2-year-old child presents with drooling and a high temperature; he is not talking and has audible inspiratory stridor. He looks miserable, with a saturation of 88% in air. Attempts to cannulate one of his veins make him very upset, and his saturation drops to 75% and stays there even with 100% high-flow oxygen.

16. A 13-year-old boy is brought to A&E with a history of difficulty in breathing. He was out with friends and smells of fireworks and smoke. He is distressed, with saturation of 80% in air; after 100% oxygen given via a mask, his saturation improves to 100%. There is inspiratory stridor as well as expiratory wheezes and stridor.

Options
A Laryngotracheomalacia
B Laryngotracheobronchitis
C Epiglotitis
D Pulmonary sling
E Laryngeal web
F Tracheal cavernous haemangioma
G Smoke inhalation
H Vascular ring
I Foreign body inhalation
J Bronchial spasms
K Bacterial tracheitis
L Acute angioedema

17–21. From the following descriptions, choose the most appropriate answer from those below:

17. An infant presents with expiratory sounds because of partial closure of the epiglottis.

18. A 3-year-old girl is seen in outpatients, and her mother describes her as struggling to breathe. She produces inspiratory noises of irregular quality and is in no respiratory distress during sleep.

19. A 4-year-old child presents to A&E with noisy breathing described by his mother as musical in sound during breathing out.

20. A 2-month-old infant is brought to hospital, as his mother is worried that he is making noises during breathing. There is a whistling sound during breathing in, which is worse when he is sleeping.

21. A 6-month-old child had an upper respiratory tract infection 2 weeks ago and is brought to hospital with a history of noisy breathing during feeding. Coarse, irregular sounds are heard during inspiration. This can be felt by putting a hand on the chest. The child is not in respiratory distress.

Options
A Stridor
B Wheezes
C Rattling
D Grunting
E Snoring
F Whistling
G Barking

22–25. The following scenarios concern pulmonary tuberculosis in children. Choose the appropriate answer from the list below:

22. A 2-year-old boy presents with a history of cough and mild fever over the last 3 weeks. His mother was treated for TB 3 years ago, and all the family have been to India on holiday this year. The Mantoux test was performed and showed an induration of 4–9 mm. He has never had BCG.

23. A 6-year-old child shows a positive Mantoux test of >10 mm induration and hilar large lymph nodes on chest X-ray.

24. A 10-year-old child was diagnosed with primary TB 4 months ago and is on treatment. He presents with fever and loss of energy and appetite. He has a persistent cough, with a large spleen and liver found on examination. There are abnormalities on auscultating his lungs. The X-ray shows diffuse mottling throughout both lung fields.

25. A 7-year-old girl has been receiving treatment for primary TB. She presents with a history of cuts on her legs and says she could not feel them on a few occasions. Her liver is 3 cm below the costal margin.

Options
A Side-effects of rifampacin
B Pneumonia on top of pulmonary TB
C Miliary TB
D Doubtful reaction to Mantoux test
E Primary tuberculosis
F Positive Mantoux test
G Side-effects of pyrazinamide
H Side-effects of isoniazid
I Pleural effusion
J Parenchymal pulmonary TB

Answers for Respiratory Medicine

1. Answer: A

Surfactant

This is dipalmitoyl phosphatidylcholine, which is a phospholipid produced by alveolar type II epithelial cells. It is enhanced by glucocorticoids, epidermal growth factors and cAMP. It is inhibited by testosterone and insulin.

2. Answer: E

Otitis media

Streptococcus pneumoniae can cause otitis media either alone or with viruses, with group Aβ haemolytic streptococci being less common. *Haemophilus influenzae* is non-typical and is responsible for causing otitis media in 2–5%. *Moraxella (Branhamella) catarrhalis* is an important organism causing otitis media. *Mycoplasma pneumoniae* is another organism that can cause otitis media. The usual symptoms are severe, with red tympanic membranes and a sometimes bulging membrane. Fever, irritability and crying can also be symptoms. Fluid can persist in the middle ear after the infection for up to 4 weeks in 50% and 12 weeks in 20%. Mastoiditis is rare, and intracranial abscesses are no longer seen since the use of antibiotics for patients with effusions and serious septic and chronic otitis media. Under the age of 2 years, children are more susceptible to a middle ear infection, for which antibiotic treatment can be justified if there is frequent, chronic otitis media or middle ear effusion and septic complications. Over 2 years of age, analgesia will be more than enough. If the membrane bursts, swabs should be taken and treated according to sensitivity. Antihistamines probably have no value, and nasal decongestants will not help. Grommet insertion is indicated for children with frequent otitis media affecting their speech.

3. Answer: E

Bronchiolitis

This is a clinical diagnosis in infants who present with coryzal symptoms, wheezes and crepitation. On clinical examination, no other findings can be found except the infant having tachypnoea, mild recession and equal air entry with marked expiratory wheezes and crepitation. There is no need to do a chest X-ray or NPA. NPA is indicated in children with chronic lung disease, congenital heart disease and immunocompromised, progressing neurological problems.

4. Answer: E

5. Answer: B

Pneumonia

Other common bacterial causes include *Mycoplasma pneumonia* and β-haemolytic streptococci, which are rare. *Klebsiella* is rare. *Chlamydia trachomatis* is common in some communities. In viral pneumonia, the clinical signs are variable, with a predominance of crackles, and very rarely there will be clinical evidence of lobar pneumonia. The radiological findings can indicate a perihilar and peribronchilar infiltrate with or without atelectasis. Bacterial pneumonia usually presents with a mild upper respiratory tract infection for several days. Infants may present with vomiting, refusal to feed, irritability and a high temperature. Grunting, tachypnoea, a slight cough and a few clinical signs may also be found. In older children, headache, fever, anorexia, restlessness, and chest pain on coughing or taking a deep breath are common, and the child is usually flushed, with tachypnoea, grunting and sometimes abdominal pain if the lower zone of the lung is affected.

6. Answer: A

7. Answer: C

8. Answer: E

9. Answer: E

Asthma management

The effectiveness of β-agonists in the first 12 months of life is not clear, but they can be given for children who present with wheezes. Wheezing may result because the bronchiolar smooth muscle is underdeveloped, the airway is small and there may be obstructions due to oedema and hypersecretion of mucous. Infants in the age group 6–12 months present with wheezes that do not affect their development and health. Inhaled steroids should be avoided in addition to regular bronchodilators. It is worthwhile to have a test dose of bronchodilators that may help to reduce the wheezes but will not stop them. This group may be benefit from using bronchodilators.

Children with recurrent wheezes associated with upper respiratory tract infections should have regular steroids, bronchodilators when needed; in acute attacks, they will need a course of 3-day oral steroids. Children who cannot tolerate exercise can benefit from using a leukotriene receptor antagonist if an increase in inhaled steroids does not help along with using bronchodilators during exercise. Children with a night cough or a cough during exercise can benefit from using a long-acting β-agonist like selmeterolol. For children with poor lung function that does not respond to regular steroids, bronchodilator inhalers may need to be investigated further. A pH study can be performed in some of these cases, as well as a sweat test.

10. Answer: D

11. Answer: E

Cystic fibrosis

Any organ could be involved as a consequence of CF. The problem will start in utero and will continue, and there is no cure at present. The future of genetic treatment is promising but still in its early stages. Infections of the lungs are the main reasons for frequent admissions to hospital. *Staphylococcus aureus* is the primary respiratory organism found, and all patients are colonized with this organism. *Pseudomonas aeruginosa* may be the initial invader. Other organisms include *Haemophilus influenzae. Moraxella (Branhamella) catarrhalis* is also isolated from a small number of patients. The source of these pathogens is unknown and could be via cross-infection. Viral infections could be blamed for starting these infections. Environmental causes such as smoking, cold weather or pollution may be the starter for the infection. Physiotherapy and physical activities are very important for children with CF and lung diseases. Co-trimoxazole, ciprofloxacin and/or flucloxacillin will be a good choice, as they are prophylactic against the above organisms if the child proves to be colonized by one of them. Aerosolized antibiotics can also be used. The regimen of a 1-week-long high dose of IV antibiotics on a monthly basis is used in some countries, and has proven to reduce the rate of admission and delay the colonization rate in these patients.

12–16. Answers:

12. B
13. F
14. A
15. C
16. G

Stridor

This is due to upper airway obstruction by various causes, all of which are mentioned above. The commonest is laryngotracheobronchitis, which is caused by viruses including parainfluenza, RSV, influenza A and B, rhinovirus and adenovirus. There is inflammatory oedema of mucosa and submucosa, causing narrowing of the subglottic area, which can cause impairment of ventilation due to small airway calibre in children. The peak incidence of croup is among 2-year-olds. Coryzal symptoms will precede breathing difficulties by 1–2 days, after which the child will start to have stridor, a barking cough and a hoarse voice. Symptoms usually develop at night and worsen by early morning. With severe airway obstruction, there is an indrawing of the suprasternal tissues and sternum during inspiration. Hypoxia may occur, and the child become agitated. Minimal disturbances, humidification, nebulized beclometasone or oral dexamethasone will help in this situation. Nebulized adrenaline will be very effective to relieve the airway obstruction temporarily if acute respiratory failure is imminent.

17–21. Answers:

> **17.** D
> **18.** E
> **19.** B
> **20.** A
> **21.** C

22–25. Answers:

> **22.** D
> **23.** E
> **24.** C
> **25.** H

Primary tuberculosis

Most children with primary TB are asymptomatic. Most are detected in a trace clinic when adults are infected and their family is screened for TB or on screening in schools. They can be divided into four groups: children with just a positive tuberculin test; children with a positive tuberculin test and radiological evidence of hilar gland enlargement; children with a positive tuberculin test, gland enlargement and lung involvement; and children with extrapulmonary TB. Miliary TB usually occurs when the organism disseminates into the bloodstream throughout the body, causing small focal lesions, including on the lungs. This may happen acutely, slowly or chronically. Beside the symptoms described in Question 24, eye examination may reveal choroidal tubercles that may be seen along the vessels and these are diagnostic. The radiological appearance is typical. Children who are not treated will develop tubercular meningitis. Drug therapy depends on the diagnosis and how extensive the lesions are. It usually lasts between 6–12 months. Drugs that are in use include isoniazid, rifampacin, pyrazinamide, streptomycin, and steroids in cases of miliary and tuberculus meningitis. In primary pulmonary tuberculosis, isonazid and rifampicin are used for 6 months and pyrazinamide for 2 months. For skin-positive contacts, isoniazid is used for 8–12 weeks. The complications of these drugs are as follows: isoniazid can cause peripheral neuritis, optic neuritis, convulsions, skin rashes and hepatomegaly; rifampicin can cause leukopenia, thrombocytopenia, orange discolouration of urine, GIT upset and hepatotoxicity; and pyrazinamide can cause hepatotoxicity, arthralgia, GIT upset, hyperuracaemia and skin rashes.

(See Phelan PD et al. *Respiratory Illness in Children*, 4th edn.)

Cardiology

BOFs

1. The following anatomical features are associated with the right atrium except:

   A The coronary sinus drains in the RA
   B The sinoatrial node presents only as a part of the conduction system in the RA
   C The septum primum is found in the RA
   D The tinea sagittalis is present in the RA
   E There are many musculi pectinati in the RA

2. The morphological anatomical features of the left ventricle (LV) is:

   A Two papillary muscles
   B Well-developed infundibulum
   C Two conduction systems
   D Fine, numerous and oblique trabeculae carneae
   E Two atrioventricular valve leaflets that are very unequal in depth

3. Which one of these syndromes is associated with total anomalous pulmonary venous return?

   A Down's
   B Turner's
   C Cat's eye
   D 49XXXXY
   E Laurence–Moon-Biedl

4. The causes of heart failure in utero include the following except:

   A Tricuspid regurgitation in Ebstein's disease
   B Arteriovenous fistula
   C Tetrology of Fallot
   D Complete heart block
   E Fetal–maternal transfusion

5. The following are true about digitalis except:

   A It increases the force and velocity of the cardiac muscle's contractility.
   B It decreases the sensitivity of the arterial baroreceptor reflex.
   C Its half-life is prolonged in children with hypothyroidism.
   D Quinidine reduces its excretion by the kidneys.
   E As a side-effect, bradycardia is more common in children than adults.

6. **Outflow obstruction from the left ventricle is characterized by the following except:**

   A It may be associated with VSD.
   B Subaortic stenosis is almost always recognized in infancy.
   C In aortic stenosis, a bicuspid aortic valve is the most common finding.
   D Subaortic valvular stenosis is more common in Williams' syndrome.
   E The diastolic pressure is lower in aortic regurgitation.

7. **The following are all causes of tachycardia with wide QRS except:**

   A SVT with BBB
   B WPW
   C Ventricular tachycardia
   D Atrial fibrillation
   E SVT with aberration

8. **The following are true about ECGs in children except:**

   A In Duchenne muscular dystrophy, the ECG will show right ventricular hypertrophy and possible SVT.
   B In tricuspid atresia, there will be a short PR interval and superior ORS axis.
   C Maternal lupus will show complete heart block in a baby.
   D Lyme disease may be associated with third degree heart block.
   E Hypothyroidism will show second-degree atrioventricular block and an absent ST segment.

9. **In ECGs, all of the following are true except:**

   A Incomplete RBBB is usually associated with RSR patterns in right pericardial leads with normal QRS.
   B The combined voltages on R and S waves in lead V4 > 35 cm indicates biventricular hypertrophy.
   C Left bundle branch block is associated with normal QRS complex and right axis deviation.
   D A peaked narrow P wave in lead II indicates right atrial enlargement.
   E Right axis deviation can be associated with RVH and left posterior hemiblock.

10. **The following are all true about echocardiography in children except:**

A In prosthetic valves, at a constant heart rate, a variation of more than a few percent in the time of opening or the duration of opening of the valve is highly suggestive of normal function.

B A greater area of disturbed flow will indicate severe valvular regurgitation.

C The velocity of flow in the regurgitant jet is not predictive of the severity of regurgitation.

D Echocardiography is superior to an X-ray in locating a pericardial effusion.

E Most cardiac lesions can be diagnosed by echocardiography at 18–20 weeks of gestation.

11. **The following are true about innocent heart murmurs except:**

A They often occur in systole.

B They are very brief, and break in the first half of systole.

C They have widespread transmission.

D Their quality is usually vibratory and musical.

E They are much louder in a supine position, with exercise and fever.

12. **In systemic hypertension, factors that can inhibit renin release include:**

A Salt loading

B Mineralocorticoids

C β blockers

D Glucagon

E Hypocalcaemia

13. **Rheumatic fever is characterized by the following except:**

A Group A β-haemolytic streptococcal pharyngitis is the main cause.

B The mitral valve is the first to be damaged.

C Aschoff bodies are found in all patients with clinical activity.

D A small percentage of patients will develop erythema marginatum.

E Sydenham's chorea is present in 50% of patients without evidence of rheumatic fever.

14. The characteristic features of Kawasaki's disease include all of the following except:

    A By the third week, there is panvasculitis of the coronary arteries, which may lead to an aneurysm.
    B A fever of 1 week or more in duration must be present even four of the other criteria are present.
    C Heart failure may occur secondary to myocarditis.
    D Coronary artery aneurysms occur in 15–25% of children with this condition.
    E Intravenous immunoglobulin in a high dose given in the first 10 days of the illness will reduce the incidence of coronary aneurysms.

15. Causes of secondary cardiomyopathy include:

    A Tyrosinaemia
    B Organic aciduria
    C Hypoparathyroidism
    D Iron overload
    E Noonan's syndrome

EMQs

16–19. From the following scenarios, choose the appropriate diagnosis about outflow obstruction of the left ventricle from the list below:

    16. A 12-year-old boy presents with a history of tiredness and lethargy. His weight is on the 3rd centile, and he looks tired and unhappy. There is an early diastolic murmur heard best on the left sternal edge and third intercostal space. The pulse pressure is high, and peripheral pulses are full and easy to feel. The ST segment is depressed on ECG, with T-wave inversion.
    17. A 1-year-old baby presents with a history of lethargy and is off his feed. The blood results showed a high calcium level with no evidence of renal calculi. There is an ejection systolic murmur at the base of the heart, radiating to the neck. Blood pressure is high at 110/65 mmHg. The infant has dysmorphic facial features.

18. A 1-week-old infant presents with difficulty in breathing and looked unwell. She was born at term, and the neonatal check showed evidence of a heart murmur that disappeared on the second day. The liver is 4 cm and palpable, and the infant is tachypnoeic and tired. She has not been able to feed for the last 12 hours. The left ventricle is huge on echocardiography, with a high left atrial pressure and clear left-to-right shunt via the foramen ovale. The PDA is open but is too small. The ST segment is depressed, with the T-wave inverted, and there is evidence of left ventricular hypertrophy. There is a systolic murmur heard at the aortic area, but no thrill and a very soft first heart sound.

19. A 10-year-old boy complains of chest pain when exercising. He fainted while running in the school grounds this morning, and was brought to hospital. The pulses are difficult to feel, with the pulse pressure being narrow. There is a thrill in the suprasternal notch, with a presystolic ejection click heard at the apex. There is an ejection systolic murmur best heard at the second right intercostal space.

Options

A Supravalvular aortic stenosis
B Critical aortic stenosis
C Subvalvular aortic stenosis
D Coarctation of the aorta
E Hypoplastic left heart syndrome
F Valvular aortic stenosis
G Aortic regurgitation
H Left coronary artery aneurysm
I Pulmonary stenosis
J Mitral stenosis
K Mitral regurgitation

20–24. The following scenarios concern arrhythmias in children. Choose the appropriate management from the list below.

20. A 7-year-old boy presents with tachycardia and looks pale. The liver is 2 cm below the right costal margin. The ECG shows a heart rate of 180 bpm with narrow QRS. The ventricular response rate varies from 2:1 to 4:1. The P wave is inverted in leads II, III and aVf.

21. A newborn baby is seen at 6 hours of age with pale colour and cold peripheries. His heart rate is above 200 bpm. The ECG has a wide QRS with a short PR interval, and a delta wave in all leads.

22. A 12-year-old boy presents with dizziness, palpitations, shortness of breath and a full feeling in the throat. The ECG shows a wide QRS with tachycardia and a dissociated P wave.

23. A 15-year-old boy was running on a school sports day. He fell and collapsed. On being taken to hospital, he was found to be tachycardic with normal QRS, T waves, ST segment and PR interval. He said he felt dizzy and that his heart was racing. The ECG was faxed to a cardiologist, who said that the QT interval was long, and echocardiography shows no structural abnormalities on his heart.

24. A 5-year-old boy was diagnosed with Refsum's syndrome. His heart rate was found to be 55 bpm, and the ECG shows ventricular ectopics with non-conducted P waves and a junctional escape rhythm at 55/min.

Options

A Pacemaker
B DC cardioversion
C IV adenosine
D IV verapamil
E Furosemide (frusemide)
F Flecainide
G Amiodarone
H Atenolol
I Quinidine
J Lidocaine (lignocaine)
K Phenytoin
L Adenosine
M Digoxin

25–28. **Choose from the following scenarios the most appropriate diagnosis from the list below:**

25. A 15-year-old presents with tachypnoea, a distended abdomen and signs of congestive heart failure. The chest X-ray shows no abnormalities. Echocardiography shows a thickening of the pericardium and limitation of cardiac motion.

26. A 7-year-old girl has just arrived from abroad and is complaining of night sweats and fever; she has lost some weight, is pale and looks tired. Her skin looks dry, her spleen is large, and she has swollen joints and a few lesions on her knuckles. There is a grade 4 systolic murmur that radiates to the neck and is best heard at the second right intercostal space.

27. A 3-month-old infant was found to have a loud ejection systolic murmur best heard at the third left intercostal space and all over the pericardium. There is no thrill, and the first and second heart sounds are within the normal range. The pulse pressure is within the normal range, and there are no added sounds. The ECG and chest X-ray are normal.

28. A 1-year-old infant was seen because of a heart murmur. There is an ejection systolic murmur loudest at the second left intercostal space, the maximal intensity being at mid-systole or later. The second heart sound is split. The pulmonary component of the second heart sound is decreased in intensity. There is an early ejection systolic click heard at the apex.

Options
A   Tetralogy of Fallot
B   Transposition of the great arteries
C   Innocent murmur
D   Aortic stenosis
E   Pulmonary stenosis
F   Constrictive pericarditis
G   Hypertrophic cardiomyopathy
H   Myocarditis
I   VSD
J   ASD
K   PDA
L   Mitral stenosis
M   Endocarditis

29–33. From the following scenarios, choose the most appropriate treatment from the list below:

29. A 6-month-old baby boy of a recently migrated family is known to have FOT that presented with cyanotic spells. He becomes short of breath and tachypnoeic, and sometimes vomits. His mother used to comfort him by holding him in an upright position with flexed knees. He improves at times, but gets tired. He was admitted to hospital with saturation in air of 85% and had one bluish episode when his saturation dropped to 66%. He is awaiting surgery.

30. A 3-month-old baby is known to have had a stridor since birth. The parents are given an assurance this will get better as he gets older. He continues to have stridor, dyspnoea and a barking cough that worsens during feeding. He has already had three upper respiratory infections. He is always choking on his food, but will then vomit and be alright. His weight is just above the 10th centile compared with his birthweight on the 50th centile. There are scattered wheezes with intercostal recession. A chest X-ray shows hyperinflation with a large thymus.

31. A newborn baby has a history of cyanosis and needs oxygen to keep his saturation at 75%. He is acidotic and very shocked. He is resuscitated, intubated and transferred to a cardiac centre. Echocardiography shows a single ventricle with no pulmonary outflow obstruction.

32. A 14-year-old boy was found unconscious in the toilets at school. He was taken to A&E, where general and systemic examinations were normal. His blood sugar is 6 mmol/l and his FBC, LFT and U&Es are normal. An ECG shows a prolonged QT interval. A 24-hour ECG shows no arrhythmia, and echocardiography is reported as normal.

33. A 13-year-old girl has suffered from constant headaches over the last 2 weeks. Occasionally, she will sleep without a headache. The problem getting worse, and no analgesia has shown any benefit. A cranial CT scan is reported as normal. Fundus examination shows papilloedema with retinal haemorrhages. Her blood pressure is 150/90 mmHg, with nothing else being noted on general or systemic examination.

Options

A DC cardioversion
B Methyldopa
C Pulmonary banding
D Correction of the vascular ring
E Blalock–Taussig correction
F Propranolol
G Magnesium sulfate
H Prostaglandin infusion
I Hydralazine
J Morphine
K Digoxin
L Calcium chloride
M Aminophylline
N Furosemide (frusemide)
O Fontan operation
P Adenosine
Q Valvoplasty

Answers for Cardiology

1. Answer: C

Anatomy of the heart

Veins draining in the RA are the inferior vena cava, constant superior vena cava and variable coronary sinus, while the veins leaving the LA are the pulmonary veins. There are few musculi pectinati in the LA. Cistera terminalis are present in the RA, but are absent from the LA. The tinea sagittalis is absent from the LA. The septum secundum is associated with the RA and the septum primum with the LA. There is no conduction system in the LA, but the sinoatrial node, atrioventricular node and bundle are on the RA.

2. Answer: B

Anatomy of the heart (ventricles)

The RV has coarse, few and straight trabeculae carneae. The papillary muscles are numerous, small, septal and free. There are three atrioventricular valve leaflets, which are equal in depth. The infundibulum is well developed, and semilunar–ventricular fibrous continuity is absent. There is one right coronary and one conduction system. Other anatomical features associated with the LV are that the paipillary muscles are large and free-wall in origin. Semilunar–atrioventricular fibrous continuity is absent. There are two coronary arteries – the left anterior descending and a branch of left coronary – and there are two conduction systems.

3. Answer: C

Total anomalous pulmonary venous return

Down's syndrome is associated with endocardial cushion, PDA, VSD and ASD. TGA, truncus arteriosus and endocardial fibroelastosis occur in children with a chromosomal aberration. TGA is not yet reported as being associated with Down's syndrome. Turner's syndrome is associated with coarctation of the aorta. 49XXXXY and 49XXXXX are associated with patent ductus arteriosus. Fetal alcohol syndrome is associated with VSD, ASD, TOF and coarctation. Williams' syndrome is associated with supravalvular aortic stenosis (most frequently), along with valvar aortic stenosis, hypoplasia of the aorta, coarctation and stenosis of peripheral blood systemic arteries (e.g. renal and peripheral pulmonary stenosis). Noonan's syndrome is associated with pulmonary valve stenosis, ASD, PDA in 10%, VSD in 10%, rarely with FOT, coarctation of the aorta, subaortic stenosis, Ebstein's malformation, complex heart defects and cardiomyopathy. Marfan's syndrome is associated with aortic arch dilation (dissection), mitral valve prolapse and dilation of the sinuses of Valsava. Trisomy 18 and trisomy 13 are also associated with many heart defects. Holt–Oram syndrome is associated with ASD. Ellis–van Creveld syndrome is associated with ASD, PDA, hypoplastic left heart syndrome, TAPVD and TGA. DiGeorge's syndrome is associated most commonly with an interrupted aortic arch, TOF and VSD, and, less frequently, with PDA and coarctation, along with other anomalies of the great vessels, especially right-sided aortic arch, and an abnormal position of the subclavian arteries.

4. Answer: C

Heart failure

Haemolytic anaemia due to RH sensitization, aplastic anaemia, SVT, atrial flutter, atrial fibrillation, ventricular tachycardia, atrioventricular valve regurgitation in the AV canal and myocarditis can cause heart failure. In addition, the following cause heart failure in neonates and infants: sepsis, HIE, hypoglycaemia, left ventricular outlet obstruction, PDA, aortopulmonary window, truncus arteriosus, VSD, single ventricle and AVSD. Rheumatic fever, viral myocarditis and bacterial endocarditis are the major causes in children. Other causes include high blood pressure, thyrotoxicoses, doxorubicin cardiomyopathy, sickle cell anaemia and cor pulmonale secondary to chronic lung disease.

5. Answer: B

Digitalis

The ionotropic effect of digitalis is usually brought about by binding to and inhibiting the Na^+/K^+ ATPase that maintains high Na^+ in myocardial cells. This will make Ca^{2+} available for contraction. Digitalis increases the sensitivity of the arterial baroreceptor reflex, resulting in an increase in vagal and a decrease in sympathetic efferent activity, which reduces the resting heart rate. Digitalis sensitivity is enhanced by hypokalaemia, hypomagnesaemia, hypocalcaemia and hyponatraemia. Hyperthyroidism will accelerate its half-life. Some antacids and neomycin will reduce its absorption. SVT and VT are less common following digitalis toxicity.

6. Answer: B

Left cardiac outflow obstruction

Left cardiac outflow obstruction can present in different ways. Infants presenting in the first 2–3 weeks of life usually have critical aortic valve stenosis, hypoplastic left heart syndrome or coarctation of the aorta. As the PDA duct starts to close, these babies will become very ill, in shock and heart failure. Emergency support is needed, and valvoplasty (which is not always successful) may save the baby's life – but valvotomy is the definitive treatment in this situation. Initial support should be given, and prostaglandin should be considered to keep the duct open, with correction of acidosis and treatment of the heart failure as an emergency measure.

Aortic stenosis normally presents and is symptomatic in teenagers with chest pain and not tolerating exercise. It is usually discovered incidentally when the murmur is found during a routine check. Aortic regurgitation very rarely occurs on its own, and is usually accompanied by aortic stenosis, TOF or VSD, or after valvoplasty for AS.

Subaortic stenosis is rarely recognized in infancy; rather, it is usually found in children of school age and older. The systolic murmur heard at the base of the heart and on echocardiography is usually helpful in diagnosing subaortic valvular stenosis. Mitral valve diseases do not cause obstruction of the left heart side. The usual investigations in suspected heart lesions include ECG, echocardiography and chest X-ray, which is not always needed. Cardiac catheterization may be needed in left hypoplastic syndrome or critical aortic stenosis. MRI can also be used in cases of supra- and subvalvular aortic stenosis, in coarctation of the aorta or in hypoplastic left heart syndrome to give the cardiologist a clear idea about the anatomy of the heart.

7. Answer: D

Tachycardia

All of these tachycardias can be terminated by DC conversion. The ECG in sinus rhythm will show BBB in SVT, with BBB, narrow PR and delta wave in WPW and normal in VT. Tachycardia usually starts and terminates very abruptly in all of these. Narrow QRS with tachycardia can be associated with atrial flutter, atrial fibrillation, SA node re-entry, junctional ectopic tachycardia, AV node re-entry, sinus tachycardia, ectopic atrial tachycardia and multifocal atrial tachycardia.

8. Answer: D

ECGs in children

In Lyme disease and Chagas' disease, a long QT can be seen. In hypocalcaemia, hypomagnesaemia and Romano–Ward and Jervell–Lange-Nielsen syndromes, interventricular conduction delay, first and/or second atrioventricular block and complete heart block will be seen. Short PR intervals are also associated with hypertrophic cardiomyopathy, WPWS, Lown–Ganongplevine syndrome and Pompe's disease. Ventricular tachycardia can be associated with hypertrophic cardiomyopathy, Romano–Ward and Jervell–Lange-Nielsen syndromes, Friedreich's ataxia, Duchenne muscular dystrophy and hyperkalaemia. SVT can associated with WPWS, myotonic dystrophy, Duchenne muscular dystrophy, Friedreich's ataxia, Lown–Ganong–Levine and Mahaim's syndromes and hypertrophic cardiomyopathy.

9. Answer: C

ECGs in children

Anterior left hemiblock is associated with left axis deviation and normal QRS, while posterior left hemiblock is associated with right axis deviation and normal QRS. Complete left bundle branch block is associated with a prolonged, slurred QRS and directs away from right chest leads.

10. Answer: A

Echocardiography

In a prosthetic valve, at a constant heart rate, a variation of more than a few percent in the time of opening or the duration of opening of the valve is highly suggestive of dysfunction. This means that there is clot development around the seating ring of the valve. Another use of echocardiography is to measure ventricular function, which can be done with a Doppler as well. Any pericardial fluid or cardiac masses can be seen on echocardiography better than on any chest X-ray films. Intraoperative use by direct application of the transducer onto the exposed heart during surgery will provide excellent images of intracardiac anatomy. Structural heart defects and valvular heart disease are the most common conditions that can be diagnosed by echocardiography.

11. Answer: C

Innocent heart murmurs

These often occur with systole – except for a venous hum, which is a continuous murmur. They are often localized, usually along the left sternal border. They are usually of grade 3, not more, and are not associated with a thrill. The intensity of the murmur changes with position, except in the case of a venous hum. Cyanosis never occurs with an innocent murmur. Still's murmur is most commonly heard in patients aged 2–7 years. It is usually a grade 3, musical, buzzing systolic ejection murmur. It is maximally heard in the third intercostal space and is louder in supine position than when sitting. It is louder with exercise, excitement and fever.

12. Answer: D

Hypertension

Other inhibitors include hyperkalaemia, hypercholesterolaemia, angiotensin II, antidiuretic hormones and A-stimulators. The stimulating factors of renin release include haemorrhage, volume depletion, hypotension, salt depletion, glucagon, parathyroid hormones, adrenocorticotrophic hormone, noradrenaline and other cathecholamines, vasodilators, diuretics, and A-stimulators. There is a long list of causes of secondary hypertension, which can be due to renal, vascular, endocrine, metabolic or neurological diseases, drugs such as steroids, heavy metals, amphetamine, contraceptives, and the use of intravenous methyldopa or cough medicine and cold preparation.

13. Answer: E

Rheumatic fever

The major manifestations of rheumatic fever include carditis, polyarthritis, erythema marginatum, Sydenham's chorea and subcutaneous nodules. Minor manifestations include fever, high ESR, elevated antistreptolysin-O-titers, abdominal pain, previous rheumatic fever, arthralgia, acute phase reaction and a prolonged PR interval. The presence of two major criteria or one major and two minor criteria indicates a high possibility of rheumatic fever. Echocardiography will be helpful in the diagnosis. The mitral valve is the first to be involved, with mitral regurgitation, apical systolic murmur and some short diastolic murmur (Carey–Coombs murmur) of mitral stenosis. Congestive cardiac failure could be the first presentation, with tachycardia, vomiting and hepatomegaly.

Treatment should be penicillin for 10 days and then prophylaxis twice a day until the patient is 21 years old. This can continue for longer, and regular review of patients is very important. Physical activity should be limited. In patients who have no active carditis salicylates can be used for pain relief and suppression of rheumatic activity.

14. Answer: B

Kawasaki's disease

The criteria for diagnosing this are a fever of 5 days (which must be present with four of the following criteria), bilateral conjunctival injection, and one of the following: injected lips, fissured lips, strawberry tongue, erythema or oedema of the hands or feet, polymorphous exanthema, and acute non-suppurative cervical lymphadenopathy.

Other symptoms include arthralgia, arthritis of small joints, sterile pyrexia, aseptic meningitis and hydrops of the gallbladder; abdominal pain and vomiting can also be presenting features, but are not diagnostic. Children with a suspected diagnosis of Kawasaki's disease should be treated with a high dose of IVIG, daily aspirin and cardiac echocardiography in the first week and again 4 weeks later. If they are then normal, no follow-up is needed, but if they are abnormal, they need cardiology follow-up and to be kept on aspirin. Laboratory investigations may show high leukocytes, a high platelet count that peaks after 4 weeks, high liver aminotransferases and a high ESR.

15. Answer: B

Cardiomyopathy

The causes of secondary cardiomyopathy include infection (viral, septicaemia, postmyocarditis or AIDS), nutritional (thiamine deficiency, kwashiorkor, pellagra or selenium deficiency), endocrine (hypo- and hyperthyroidism, phaeochromocytoma, infant of a diabetic mother or hypoglycaemia), neuromuscular (Friedrich's ataxia or Duchenne musculur dystrophy), lupus erythematosus, drugs (anthracyclines, steroids or catecholamines), Beckwith–Wiedemann syndrome, multiple lentigines, epidermolysis bullosa, Turner's syndrome, Kawasaki's disease and rheumatic fever. The primary causes include many metabolic disorders (lysosomal enzyme deficiency, fatty acids, glucose utilization, protein metabolism, pyruvate metabolism, citric acid cycle, etc.).

16–19. Answers:

16. H
17. A (Williams' syndrome)
18. B
19. F
See answer to Question 6.

20–24. Answers:

20. A (atrial flutter), **B, L:** Other drugs that can be used if the above fail include quinidine, flecainide and amiodarone, to terminate the arrhythmia, slow the atrial conduction velocity and lengthen the atrial refractory periods.

21. C (SVT with WPW), **F:** Another intervention that can be used is DC cardioversion if the child is very sick and not stable. Verapamil is contraindicated in patients with SVT and WPWs. Digoxin can be used if others fail as a maintenance drug, but not in WPWs patients, as it may accelerate the rate of atrial impulse conduction in accessory connection, as with verapamil. Surgical aberration is the ultimate treatment for children by the age of 10 years who do not respond or have been on long-term treatment.

22. B (VT): If there is no response to DC cardioversion, IV lidocaine as a bolus should be administered, followed by an infusion. The second choice is procainamide. If the VT is secondary to digoxin toxicity, phenytoin can be used. There is no place for verapamil and digoxin in the emergency treatment of VT. Ventricular pacing can be done if there is no response to medication.

23. A (prolonged QT syndrome): Initial treatment with propanolol can be given. Other drugs that can be used include phenytoin and lidocaine. For long-term therapy, if no pacemaker is required, mexiletine, phenytoin can be used.

Causes of prolonged QT are Ramono–Ward syndrome, Jervell–Lange-Nielsen syndrome, class I and III antiarrhythmic drugs, phenothiazines, tricyclic antidepressants, organophosphates, pentamidine, complete heart block, dilated myopathy, sick sinus syndrome, hypocalcaemia, hypomagnesaemia, hypokalaemia, HIV infection and CNS injuries.

24. A (third-degree heart block).

25–28. Answers:

25. F
26. M
27. I (small VSD)
28. E

Congenital heart diseases

Congenital heart diseases can be cyanotic or acyanotic. Cyanotic heart diseases may present from the first day of life or later on up to 1 year of age. These should be corrected early to prevent the development of pulmonary hypertension, which can be difficult to correct. The commonest congenital acyanotic heart disease is a ventricular septal defect (VSD), which can be solitary or associated with other lesions such as TOF, TOGA or Avcanal. VSD is more common in premature babies and stillborns. Between 15% and 50% of VSDs close spontaneously, mainly in first 6 months of life. Echocardiography is the tool for diagnosis. VSD is due to a delay in the closure of the interventricular septum beyond the first 7 weeks of intrauterine life, and the cause is unknown. The sibling of an affected child will have an increased risk of VSD, but children of parents with VSD will be at low risk, as it is not a prominent feature. There are many types of membranous (most common at 75%) VSDs, which is a small area immediately adjacent to and under the aortic valve on the left side, contagious to the septal leaflet of the tricuspid valve on the right side and overlapping a small segment of the right atrium. Muscular VSDs can be located in any part of the apical, mid, anterior or posterior muscular septum and are often multiple. Both muscular and membranous VSDs close spontaneously more frequently than others. Infundibular (subpulmonary) VSDs are located under the pulmonary valve when viewed from the right and under the aortic valve when viewed from the left. The adjacent aortic valve cusps prolapse into the left ventricle with aortic regurgitation. The endocardial cushion type is associated with Down's syndrome. It is located beneath the tricuspid valve, extending to the tricuspid valve ring, and occupies the area where an atrioventricularis communis opening is normally found. Large defects are usually present, with congestive heart failure and a murmur. Initially, the baby is fine, but will then develop tachypnoea and tachycardia prior to heart failure. Growth failure and a malnourished appearance are common problems. The heart murmur of a VSD is influenced by the size of the VSD, the pressure difference between the two ventricles and the amount of left-to-right shunt. If the shunt is from right to left, there will be no murmur. The smaller the defect, the louder the murmur.

29–33. Answers:

29. F
30. D
31. H, J
32. F
33. B, G, I

Gastroenterology

BOFs

1. Causes of upper GIT bleeding include:

   A Mallory–Weiss tear
   B Meckel's diverticulum
   C Haemolytic uraemic syndrome
   D Cow's milk intolerance
   E Intussusception

2. All of the following are true about *Helicobacter pylori* except:

   A It can cause antral gastritis only.
   B It usually presents with melaena.
   C The organism can be visualized at the mucosal surface on silver and Giemsa staining.
   D The CLO test is 97% sensitive and 98% specific.
   E Gastritis is less common in children than in adults.

3. All of the following are causes of painless lower GIT bleeding in children except:

   A Inflammatory bowel disease
   B Arteriovenous malformation
   C Cow's milk protein intolerance
   D Juvenile polyps
   E Peutz–Jeghers syndrome

4. All of the following are causes of rectal prolapse in children except:

   A Solitary rectal prolapse syndrome
   B Acute diarrhoeal illness
   C Rectal polyps
   D Inflammatory bowel disease
   E Constipation

5. The following are causes of occult GIT bleeding in children except:

   A Vascular anomalies
   B Haemangioma
   C Non-*Helicobacter* gastritis
   D Oesophagitis
   E Intussusception

6. The following are true of gastro-oesophageal reflux (GOR) except:

   A Oesophageal acid exposure is limited by swallowing.
   B Oesophageal pH increases abruptly following swallowing.
   C Trypsin and pepsin can be found in refluxing fluid.
   D Poor mucosal defence may cause oesophagitis as a result of GOR.
   E Lower oesophageal sphincter tone is lost indefinitely during episodes of reflux (lower oesophageal relaxation).

7. The following are common organic causes of recurrent abdominal pain except:

   A Coeliac disease
   B Pancreatic insufficiency
   C Peutz–Jeghers syndrome
   D Carbohydrate malabsorption
   E Giardiasis

8. In inflammatory bowel disease, the following are true except:

   A Abdominal pain is more commonly associated with ulcerative colitis (UC).
   B Diarrhoea is more commonly associated with Crohn's disease (CD).
   C Weight loss can happen in both UL and CD.
   D Fever is more commonly associated with CD.
   E Bleeding per rectum occurs less frequently with CD.

9. The following are true about the pathology of CD and UC except:

   A In UC, inflammation is limited to the mucosa of the rectum and colon.
   B In CD, the presence of non-caseating granulomas is limited to disease of the small intestine.
   C In CD, submucosal and transmural changes are universal.
   D In UC in children, pancolitis is a more common presentation than in adults.
   E Crypt abscesses are more commonly associated with UC.

10. **The following are true about the management of UC and CD except:**

    A Nutritional therapy is effective in inducing remission in CD, but not in UC.

    B Polymeric feeds contain whole protein and are better tolerated orally than elemental feeds.

    C 5-Aminosalicylates are effective as monotherapy to induce remission in patients with CD.

    D Azathioprine and 6-mercaptopurine are effective in both CD and UC.

    E Systemic corticosteroids are the mainstay of remission induction in UC and CD.

11. **All of the following are true about gastrin secreted from the antrum except:**

    A It stimulates secretion of pepsinogen.

    B It stimulates secretion of pancreatic enzymes.

    C It increases lower oesophageal sphincter tone.

    D It stimulates secretion of gastric acid.

    E It increases gastric motility.

12. **The following are true about digestion and absorption of food except:**

    A In the luminal phase of carbohydrate hydrolysis, α-amylases are limited to breaking α1–4 linkages.

    B Sucrase hydrolyses sucrose to glucose and fructose.

    C Trypsin will cleave pancreatic proenzymes.

    D Mixed micelles are formed by interaction of fatty acids and mono-glycerides with bile acids.

    E Free amino acids are absorbed faster in the jejunum than di- or tripeptides are.

13. **The following formula milks have MCT except:**

    A Nutramigen

    B Pregestimil

    C Prejomin

    D Aptamil

    E Peptijunior

14. **The following formula milks have reduced lactose content except:**

    A Enfamil

    B Galactomin

    C Similac

    D Prejestimil

    E Pre-aptamil

15. Oral hydration solution is characterized by the following except:

   A Its aim is to correct acid–base and electrolyte disturbances.
   B The sodium content of Dioralyte is 60 mmol per sachet.
   C The glucose content of Dioralyte is 50 g/l.
   D The overall osmolarity of ORS is 270–310 mosmol/l.
   E The citrate content of Dioralyte is 20 mmol/l.

16. The following investigations are likely to help in cows' milk protein intolerance except:

   A Stool pH
   B Skin prick test
   C Small-bowel biopsy
   D Eosinophilic count
   E Total IgE

17. In a differential diagnosis of cows' milk protein intolerance, one should exclude:

   A Constipation
   B Coeliac disease
   C Gastroesophageal reflux
   D Campylobacter infection
   E HIV infection

18. In food intolerance, which of the following is the symptom least likely to occur?

   A Vomiting
   B Abdominal pain
   C Steatorrhoea
   D Diarrhoea
   E Urticaria

19. The feature favouring a diagnosis of bulimia rather than anorexia is:

   A Bodyweight is maintained at least 15% below that expected.
   B Bodyweight is maintained at least 10% below that expected.
   C There is body image distortion.
   D Pubertal events are delayed.
   E There is amenorrhoea due to problems in the hypothalamic–pituitary–gonadal axis.

20. The feature favouring a diagnosis of anorexia nervosa rather than bulimia is:

A Weight loss self-induced by avoidance of fattening food
B Self-induced purging
C Excessive exercise
D Binge eating
E Use of appetite suppressants and diuretics

21. The following investigations can usually help in diagnosing pancreatic exocrine insufficiency disorders except:

A Sweat test
B Bone survey
C Small-bowel biopsy
D Barium swallow and follow-through
E Serum immunoreactive trypsin

22. Features associated with Shwachman–Diamond syndrome include the following except:

A Thrombocytopenia
B Metaphyseal dysplasia
C Focal biliary cirrhosis
D HbF present in 80% of patients
E Diabetes mellitus

23. In infantile pyloric stenosis:

A Most cases are sporadic.
B In the UK, it is more common than cystic fibrosis.
C It is more common in children with blood group A.
D The obstruction is due to fibrotic changes in the pyloric muscle.
E The symptoms always start between 2 weeks and 2 months of age.

24. Regarding *Helicobacter pylori* (HP) all of the following are true except:

A In developing countries, it is mostly acquired during childhood.
B If acquired during childhood, most children will clear it due to a mounting host response.
C HP tends to colonize the stomach more than the proximal duodenum.
D It spreads by the oral–oral and faecal–oral routes.
E For diagnosis, the [^{13}C]urea breath test is more specific than serology showing positive IgG to HP in the serum.

25. In gastro-oesophageal reflux (GOR) all of the following are false accept:

A GOR is less common than infantile pyloric stenosis in babies less than 3 months of age.

B It is commonly associated with developmental delay.

C In most cases nowadays, the diagnosis is made by a 24-hour pH study.

D Chronic respiratory disease exacerbates GOR.

E In the management of significant GOR, the prone position with head raised is recommended.

26. In coeliac disease, all of the following are true except:

A The enteropathy involves different parts of the small intestine in a patchy pattern.

B There is an increased incidence among children with Down's syndrome.

C There is an increased incidence among children with insulin-dependent diabetes mellitus.

D The majority of children present with chronic diarrhoea and poor weight gain.

E Treatment with a gluten-free diet is lifelong.

27. The following are true except:

A There is an increased incidence of infection with *Giardia lamblia* in children with isolated IgA deficiency.

B There is an increased incidence of infection with *Giardia lamblia* in children with common variable immunodeficiency disease.

C Cows' milk protein intolerance does not affect strictly breastfed babies.

D The natural history of cows' milk protein intolerance is one of spontaneous remission.

E In short-gut syndrome, there is an increased risk of peptic ulcers if a large length of the jejunum is resected.

EMQs

28–32. For the following scenarios in children presenting with GIT bleeding, choose from the list below the most appropriate investigations:

28. A 14-year-old boy presents with a long history of jaundice, maelena and poor weight gain. The liver is about 3 cm below the right costal margin. His ALT is 180 iu/l, bilirubin is 300 mmol/l (with 250 mmol/l conjugated). Alk phos is 600 iu/l and albumin is 26 g/l.

29. A 9-year-old girl presents with recurrent abdominal pain, maelena and vomiting from time to time. Upper GIT endoscopy shows gastritis and a small amount of bleeding from the stomach. A biopsy is taken and shows gastritis with the possibility of an organism.
30. An 18-month-old infant presents with maelena, vomiting and diarrhoea. He has been weaned off breast milk and put on formula milk over the last 3 months. He is otherwise well. Colonoscopy shows mucosal erythema and procto-colitis. Eosinophilic filtration and aphthous ulceration are seen on histology.
31. A 3-year-old girl presents with massive frank painless bleeding. Her Hb has dropped to 6.7 g/dl. She is transfused. Her upper and lower GIT endoscopy are normal. She says that her abdomen is hurting her from time to time around the umbilicus when she eats any spicy foods. The abdomen is soft and not tender, and there is no organomegaly. Abdominal ultrasound shows no abnormalities and the stool culture is negative for bacteria and protozoa.
32. A 4-year-old boy presents with painless rectal bleeding over the last 5 days. His mother reports that his anus looks red and fresh blood has been seen. His abdomen is soft and abdominal X-ray shows no evidence of constipation. His ESR is <10 and his Hb is 9.8 g/dl. The stool shows no organisms. His father died at the age of 40 years with a large-bowel malignancy.

Options
A Upper GIT endoscopy with biopsies
B Abdominal ultrasound
C Barium swallow and follow-through
D Liver biopsy
E Coagulation screen
F Viral serology for hepatitis B, C, D, E
G Colonoscopy with biopsy
H [^{99m}Tc]pertechnetate scan
I Rast test for IgE (dairy products)
J CLO test
K Mesenteric angiography
L ESR
M Stool culture for bacteria and protozoa
N Abdominal X-ray
O Abdominal CT
P Abdominal MRI
Q Laparotomy
R Video capsule endoscopy

33–36. For the following scenarios, choose from the list below the most appropriate diagnoses:

33. An 8-year-old girl presents with a history of recurrent abdominal pain, which she says gets better when she opens her bowels. She always feels that she wants to go to the toilet again to empty her bowels. She feels bloated, and her abdomen is distended most of time according to her mother. Upper GIT endoscopy is normal and a barium swallow shows no abnormalities. Skin prick tests for dairy, eggs, fish and various vegetables are normal. Her examination shows no abnormalities apart from generalized tenderness and a reluctance to allow anyone to touch her abdominal wall. Abdominal ultrasound, biopsies from the large intestine and abdominal MRI show no abnormalities.

34. An 11-year-old boy complains of persisting pain in his upper abdomen. He says that he feels sick most of the time. His pain most of the time is relieved by food. It occurs before meals and when he is hungry. He wakes almost every night with abdominal pain and his mother has to give him a sugary drink, which helps him to sleep. Upper GIT endoscopy shows red mucosa with a few small bleeds on the antrum of the stomach. He is started on antacids and omeprazole 10 mg twice daily for 6 weeks, which helps him considerably.

35. A 7-year-old girl presents with recurrent daily abdominal pain. Over the last 3 months she has been unable to attend school while under investigation. The pain is periumbilical and never wakes her up at night. Not eating or drinking can make it worse. She is investigated with blood test, skin prick test, and abdominal ultrasound. Hyoscine butylbromide and dicycloverine (dicyclomine) hydrochloride help on some days. Nothing is found on physical examination, and her bowel movements are regular. Her mother said that the problem started after she had gastroenteritis when she was 6 years old.

36. A 6-year-old girl presents with recurrent abdominal pain lasting between 4 hours and 2 days on two occasions. She always becomes pale and feels sick. She says that this is sometimes associated with headache and pain in her eyes. Her examination shows no abnormalities and a blood test including FBC, LFT and ESR is normal, as is abdominal ultrasound. She is well between episodes, which occur 2–3 weeks apart.

Options
A Gastric ulcer
B Gastro-oesophageal reflux
C Giardiasis
D Abetalipoproteinaemia
E Chronic renal failure
F Polycystic renal disorder
G Liver fibrosis
H Hypersplenism
I Irritable bowel syndrome
J Abdominal migraine
K Cholecystitis
L Inflammatory bowel disease
M Functional abdominal syndrome
N Lactose intolerance
O Aerophagia
P Coeliac disease

Answers for Gastroenterology

1. Answer: D

2. Answer: A

Helicobacter pylori

H. pylori is also a major cause of antral gastritis and peptic ulcers. In children, ulcers are usually present in the duodenum rather than the stomach. It usually presents as melaena, but occasionally with vomiting. Upper GIT endoscopy is the appropriate diagnostic tool for this, and a biopsy must be taken from the antral part of the stomach. *H. pylori* is a urea-splitting organism, and in the CLO test, the release of ammonia turns the orange test medium pink within a few hours if the organism is present in a biopsy. Endoscopic treatment of ulcers is indicated if they are actively bleeding. This can be done by injecting saline or adrenaline or by using thermal therapy at the bleeding site. The recurrence rate for bleeding is less than 3%. Medical treatment consists of a 1-week course of an acid suppressant (either a proton pump inhibitor such as omeprazole or the H_2 receptor antagonist ranitidine) together with two antibiotics (generally amoxicillin plus either clarithromycin or metronidazole, although the combination of clarithromycin and metronidazole may be used in certain cases). Full details of the recommended regimes are given in the BNF for Children, page 56. 2005 edition.

3. Answer: A

Painful lower GIT bleeding

Painful lower GIT bleeding with frank blood may be caused by necrotizing enterocolitis, intussusception, anal fissure, rectal varices, haemorrhoids, rectal prolapse, infectious colitis, intestinal necrosis, solitary rectal ulcer, haemangioma and inflammatory bowel disease.

4. Answer: D

Rectal prolapse

This usually occurs in infants, and may be associated with rectal bleeding. Constipation is the most common cause; this can lead to repetitive straining, which can cause rectal prolapse. Other causes include cystic fibrosis, local anatomical problems, surgery on the anal area and neurological problems. The solitary rectal prolapse syndrome is usually present, with constipation, bleeding, localized perianal pain, mucus discharge and straining with tenesmus. It is usually resolved when the constipation is treated. The cause of rectal prolapse should be found and treated.

5. Answer: E

There are many causes of occult bleeding in the GIT. For the upper GIT tract, these include peptic ulcer and Meckel's diverticulum. In the lower GIT, causes include cow's milk protein intolerance. Occult bleeding anywhere in the GIT can be due to vascular anomalies, inflammatory bowel disease, polyps, intestinal necrosis and haemangioma. Investigations should include upper and lower GIT endoscopy.

6. Answer: E

Gastro-oesophageal reflux

The following factors can contribute to GOR:

- defective oesophageal peristalsis
- poor oesophageal mucosal defence
- content of the refluxing fluid
- inappropriate relaxation of lower oesophageal sphincter tone, which can transiently lead to a phenomenon called transient lower oesophageal sphincter relaxation
- anatomical malformation (e.g. hiatus hernia)
- content and size of meals
- delayed gastric emptying and abnormal motility

7. Answer: B

Recurrent abdominal pain

Recurrent abdominal pain can be defined as pain of more than 3 months duration with a recurrent nature. In two-thirds of cases, no cause can be found, and the condition is labelled as functional. The development of investigative procedures such as endoscopy has helped to find more causes and aided their treatment. Inflammatory bowel disease and gallbladder, liver and renal tract disease can cause recurrent abdominal pain in children. Other causes include gastritis, GOR, gastric and duodenal ulcers with *Helicobacter pylori* infection, and non-steroidal anti-inflammatory drugs. Half of patients with non-functional abdominal pain will have features of irritable bowel syndrome, including abdominal pain relieved by opening the bowels, more frequent and looser stools at the onset of pain, passage of mucus, a sensation of incomplete emptying of the bowel, and a feeling of bloating.

8. Answer: B

9. Answer: B

10. Answer: C

Inflammatory bowel disease

The mean age group of children with IBD is 12 years, with 25% of IBD cases occurring in the paediatric age group. The causes of IBD are still unknown. Many theories suggest a multifactorial aetiology, including genetic, environmental and immunological causes. The presentation in UC is usually with bloody diarrhoea, which can be intermittent, Tenesmus is common, and abdominal pain tends to be prior to opening the bowels when inflammation has reached the sigmoid colon. In CD, symptoms are more subtle, due to diffuse and diverse anatomical localization. Abdominal pain, diarrhoea and weight loss is the classical presentation of CD. Systemic symptoms such as anorexia, lethargy, pyrexia, arthralgia, arthritis and erythema nodosum are more common with CD than with UC, as are growth failure and pubertal delay. More than 50% of children with CD will have abnormalities around the anal area. In the case of a clinical suspicion of IBD, upper and lower GIT endoscopy with biopsies should be performed without delay. UC is usually limited to the large bowel and is extensive in children as pancolitis. The microscopic features of UC are limited to the mucosa and are continuous from rectum to colon. There is intense neutrophilic infiltration in the mucosa, with goblet cell depletion, crypt distortion and crypt abscesses. CD can affect any part of the gastrointestinal system, from mouth to anus. It is also more extensive in children, with the ileum and colon being mostly affected. The lesions are usually focal and asymmetrical, with transmural extension. Non-caseating granulomas and fissuring ulceration may be present. Treatment can involve nutritional therapy, drugs and surgery. Nutritional therapy is more effective in producing remission in CD than in UC. There are two types: an elemental diet and a polymeric diet, both of which can produce remission if given for 6 weeks (no other diet should be given). A polymeric diet is superior to an elemental diet. Drugs include 5-aminosalicylates (which can prolong remission in cases of UC), corticosteroids, and azathioprine and its metabolite 6-mercaptopurine (which should be combined with steroids or nutritional therapy for 3 months). Surgery is usually avoided in CD, but can be curative in UC. It may be performed in cases where medical treatment has failed, or the patient has become steroid-dependent.

11. Answer: A

12. Answer: B

Digestion and absorption of food

The digestion and absorption of carbohydrates have two phases. The initial stage of carbohydrate hydrolysis is the luminal phase, which takes place in the duodenum under the action of pancreatic α-amylases. This involves the breakdown of α1–4 linkages only; sucrose and lactose are not hydrolysed. The mucosal phase occurs in the small intestine, where enzymes hydrolyse residual sugars and α1–6-linked carbohydrate molecules. Following this, monosaccharides are transported to enterocytes. Glucose is absorbed via Na–monosaccharide cotransporters.

Proteins start to be digested in the stomach by proteinases produced by gastric cells in the form of the proenzyme pepsinogen and activated by the low gastric pH. About one-third of protein hydrolysis occurs in the duodenum. Several pancreatic proteinases are also involved in the hydrolysis. Di- and tripeptides are absorbed more rapidly in the jejunum than are free amino acids.

Fat digestion usually starts in the mouth and stomach; an emulsion is produced, and small amounts of triglycerides are hydrolysed in the stomach. When the acidic stomach contents reach the duodenum, secretin is released from the duodenal mucosa into the portal circulation. This stimulates the pancreas to produce and release bicarbonate, lipase and colipase into the duodenum. Lipase and colipase act at the surface of particles and hydrolyse tri- and monoglycerides and fatty acids. The formation of mixed micelles is the last step, involving interaction of fatty acids and monoglycerides with bile acids. Vitamins D, E and K require these micelles for their absorption.

The following hormones are produced by the GIT:

- gastrin
- secretin, which is secreted by the duodenum, inhibiting gastrin secretion, stimulating pancreatic water and bicarbonate secretion and increasing insulin release
- gastric inhibitory peptide, which is secreted by the duodenum and jejunum and acts on the stomach, inhibiting secretin and gastrin secretion
- cholecystokinin, which is secreted by the duodenum and acts on the pancreas, inhibiting GIT motility, stimulating secretion of pancreatic enzymes, stimulating contraction of the gallbladder and slowing gastric emptying
- somatostatin, which is secreted by the antrum, inhibiting gastrin and motilin secretion, inhibiting pancreatic secretion and decreasing GIT motility
- motilin, which is secreted by the antrum and duodenum, stimulating gastric emptying and increasing GIT motility

13. Answer: D

14. Answer: E

Formula milks

Formulas containing hydrolysed protein and MCT:

• Hydrolysed protein milk	MCT milk
• Peptide 0–2 (soya and meat protein)	2.6% MCT, 97.4% LCT
• Nutramigen (casein)	2.9% MCT, 97.1% LCT
• Peptijunior (whey-based protein)	50% MCT, 50% LCT
• Prejestimil (casein)	55% MCT, 45% LCT
• Prejomin (soya and protein collagens)	6% MCT, 94% LCT
• Aptamil (whole milk)	Vegetable oil and egg

Protein-based milks can be extensively hydrolysed or partially hydrolysed. The protein can be cows' milk (whey and casein), soya or collagen derived from meat. The protein is hydrolysed by proteolyic enzymes, heat treatment and ultrafiltration to reduce the whole protein to short-chain peptides. Casein-based formulas are the least allergenic, while whey-based formulas have large peptides and are more allergenic. Extensively hydrolysed formulas are free of lactose, while partially hydrolysed formulas contain lactose. Extensively hydrolysed formulas contain MCTs, while partially hydrolysed formulas have a fat content similar to that of whole milk.

Formulas with reduced lactose content are based on cows' milk and may be whey- or casein-dominant. The fat source is either vegetable oils or a mixture of butterfat and vegetable oil. The lactose is replaced by glucose polymers or maltodextrin with a residual lactose content of 10 mg/100 ml. Because of the low lactose content, these are not good for treatment of galactosaemia, where a soya-based formula is preferred.

Soya formulas are used for infants with cows' milk protein intolerance. Protein soya is supplemented with L-methionine, l-carnitine and taurine. The fat content comes from vegetables and the carbohydrates from starch. Soymilk is free of milk protein, lactose and gluten.

Breast milk fortifiers are for low-birthweight, sick or premature babies. These can be added to breast milk, but the latter will not retain its anti-infective properties. Nutriprem and SMA are breast milk fortifiers, while Enfamil is a human milk fortifier.

15. Answer: C

Oral hydration fluid

Contents	Dioralyte	WHO rehydration fluid	Homemade ORS (5 g salt and 25 g glucose per 1000 ml water)
Sodium	60 mmol/l	90 mmol/l	85 mmol/l
Potassium	20 mmol/l	20 mmol/l	0
Chloride	60 mmol/l	80 mmol/l	85 mmol/l
Base	(citrate) 20 mmol/l	(citrate) 30 mmol/l	0
Glucose	16 g/l	20 g/l	92 mmol/l

ORS is used as a treatment in diarrhoea to minimize dehydration and to correct acid–base and electrolyte disturbances. The most important ingredients are sodium and glucose. The recommended sodium content for a well-nourished child is 45–50 mmol/l (90 mmol/l for malnourished children). Carbohydrates should not exceed 25 g/l. Inclusion of potassium and a base is not necessary; these can be supplied in the form of foods such as bananas. The inclusion of starch has some benefit in children with secretory diarrhoea and for older children. It should be mixed with boiling water before use.

16. Answer: A

17. Answer: B

Cows' milk protein-sensitive enteropathy

This can be preceded by acute gastroenteritis, or it may come on suddenly. It appears as an allergic reaction with a positive family history of atopy. β-Lactoglobulin is the most common cause of this allergic reaction, but many proteins (up to 20) can be involved. It usually mimics prolonged gastroenteritis, and can include vomiting and large volumes of stools containing mucus and microscopic or macroscopic blood. Failure to thrive is the main feature, and children switched to soymilk may continue to have the same symptoms, as 25% of children allergic to cows' milk are also allergic to soymilk. Colic may present early and may continue.

Skin prick testing will give immediate results, but a radioallergosorbent test (RAST) can produce false-positive as well as false-negative results, so will fail to identify the problem. If the small intestine is affected, a small-bowel biopsy will show patchy enteropathy with chronic inflammation (infiltrate lymphocytes and eosinophils). Eosinophilia, elevated IgE, low IgA and reduced C3 with possible iron deficiency anaemia may also be seen. Stools will show Charcot–Leyden crystals (eosinophils) and the pH will be normal. Other causes of diarrhoea to be excluded are lactose malabsorption, coeliac disease, giardiasis, irritable bowel syndrome, enteritis, intestinal lymphangiectasia and immunodeficiency syndromes.

Infants on breast milk will not have a problem, but the mother should avoid dairy products. The baby should be switched to hydrolysed milk protein (Nutramigen, Pregestimil and peptide-based milks), other milks from humans, goats or sheep, or feed based on soymilk. Reintroduction of cows' milk can be done after 2 years, but a skin prick test should be performed prior to this.

18. Answer: C

Food intolerance

In a group of 62 children with food intolerance, the percentages of symptoms arising were as follows:

Vomiting 47%	Diarrhoea 41%	Crying 35%
Failure to thrive 31%	Eczema 22%	Abdominal pain 19%
Wheeze 19%	Urticaria 18%	Other rashes 13%
Mood alteration 12%	Angioneurotic oedema 10%	Flatulence 10%
Abdominal distension 7%	Steatorrhoea 3%	

19. Answer: B

20. Answer: B

Eating disorders

	Anorexia	Bulimia
Age of onset	Early or late adolescence	Early or late adolescence
% below normal weight	<15%	>10%
Binge eating	Occasional	Frequently
Behaviour	Fast foods and forbidden foods	Binging on forbidden foods
Disturbance of endocrine system	Yes	Yes
Behaviour	Self-induced purging, excessive exercise, use of appetite suppressants and diuretics	Self-induced vomiting, misuse of laxatives, diuretics, enemas, fasting, excessive exercise

The full recovery rate in women with anorexia nervosa is 33%, whereas that in bulimia is 75% over a period of 90 months. Partial recovery is much better in bulimic patients. One-third of women will relapse after recovery in both bulimia and anorexia. Cognitive–behavioural therapy is the approach to managing both of these groups of patients. Antidepressants can be helpful, especially in bulimic anorexic patients.

21. Answer: C

22. Answer: C

Pancreatic exocrine insufficiency disorders

The most common pancreatic exocrine insufficiency disorder is cystic fibrosis (CF), followed by Shwachman–Diamond syndrome, and, very rarely, trypsinogen, enterokinase, lipase, combined lipase–colipase and pancreatic amylase enzyme deficiencies. Manifestations of Shwachman–Diamond syndrome include short stature, metaphyseal dysplasia, cup-shaped ribs, hypoplasia of the iliac bones, susceptibility to infection, anaemia with 80% HbF, thrombocytopenia, pancreatic exocrine abnormalities, myelodysplastic syndrome in 33%, skin disorders (eczema and ichthyosis), hepatic dysfunction and cardiac failure. It may present with Hirschprung's disease, diabetes mellitus and hepatosplenomegaly. Humoral immunodeficiency is common. Fat loss decreases with age because of the increase in lipase secretion. Learning difficulties are reported in 25% of patients. A sweat test to exclude CF must be performed, and faecal fat studies is important, as well as a pancreatic stimulation test to measure levels of trypsin, amylase and lipase. Bone surveys should be performed to identify skeletal abnormalities not found in any other pancreatic exocrine insufficiency disorders. HbF is found in 80% of patients, and IgA and IgM are low, with low thymine. A white cell function test should be performed to locate the defect in neutrophils. Bone marrow aspiration should be performed to determine whether the patient suffers from myelodysplastic syndrome. Enzyme replacement is important, and can be lifelong.

23. Answer: B

Infantile pyloric stenosis

Infantile pyloric stenosis is characterized by the onset of projectile vomiting in infants between the 2nd and 4th weeks of age, although earlier and later onset up until the age of 4 months is not rare. It has an incidence of about 3/1000 infants, with a strong familial pattern, and is more common in boys (M:F = 4:1). For uncertain reasons, the pyloric muscle hypertrophies and thickens, causing progressive obstruction at the outlet of the stomach. The typical symptom is projectile vomiting, which can gradually lead to dehydration. Typical signs are visible gastric peristalsis and a palpable pyloric tumour in the upper abdomen to the right of the midline. The typical cases show hypokalaemic metabolic alkalosis, and the diagnosis can be made clinically by observing a test feed. Otherwise, it can be made by an ultrasound scan, although in the early stages the result can be equivocal. The management includes correction of any fluid or electrolyte disturbances and surgical pyloromyotomy. Interestingly, infantile pyloric stenosis is noticeably less common in infants with blood group A.

24. Answer: B

Helicobacter pylori

In developing countries, due to poor hygiene and overcrowding, about 80% of the population will acquire HP by adolescence. In the majority of cases, the infection will persist despite a mounting host response. HP colonizes the duodenum only after a long time of colonizing the stomach and causing changes in the gastric mucosa.

The urea breath test has about 90% sensitivity and 100% specificity, while positive serology has sensitivity and specificity around 90%. The other ways of making the diagnosis are a trial of treatment and obtaining a culture specimen by endoscopy. Full details of the recommended regimes are given in *BNF for Children*, page 56. 2005 edition.

25. Answer: D

Gastro-oesophageal reflux

GOR is a very common physiological/pathological phenomenon in infancy: almost all babies have some degree of GOR. The reflux of food back up from the stomach is normally prevented by many mechanisms, including three types of oesophageal peristalsis, the anatomy of the oesophagus in relation to the stomach and the diaphragm, and the presence of upper and lower oesophageal sphincters. Disturbance of any of these can lead to the development of GOR. For example, children with cerebral palsy have very poor peristaltic activities, and children with a hiatus hernia have disturbed anatomy. The diagnosis is usually made clinically. A 24-hour pH study can quantify the degree of GOR. Treatment options include positioning in the left lateral position, prokinetic agents such as domperidone, feed thickeners and H_2 antihistamines. Surgical intervention is required in some severe cases. The prone position is not recommended, as it increases the risk of sudden infant death syndrome.

26. Answer: A

Coeliac disease

The enteropathy involves predominantly the proximal small intestine in a diffuse pattern. Many coeliac children present with other symptoms, such as constipation, anaemia and short stature. In fact, the diagnosis sometimes is made in asymptomatic siblings.

27. Answer: C

If the mother's diet includes cows' milk, the baby could get cows' milk protein intolerance, as the cows' milk protein can be excreted in the breast milk. Although most children with isolated IgA deficiency are asymptomatic, they have an increased incidence of infection with *Giardia lamblia*. The jejunum is responsible for the digestion of gastrin, and so resecting a large length of the jejunum can cause hypergastrinaemia and peptic ulceration.

28–32. Answers:

28. B, D, E, F (oesophageal varices secondary to portal hypertension)
29. J (gastritis with gastric bleeding secondary to *H. pylori* infection)
30. I, L, M (Cow's milk intolerance)
31. H (Meckel's diverticulum)
32. G (Familial adenomatous polyposis)

GIT bleeding

In babies younger than 1 month, GIT bleeding can be due to infection or necrotizing enterocolitis. Trauma is very unlikely. In infants up to 2 years old, it can be due to cow's milk intolerance, intussusception, constipation with anal fissure, intermittent malrotation or partial volvulus, infection, intestinal necrosis, or rectal prolapse. At ages above 2 years, all of the above causes are possible, as well as rectal varices, haemorrhoids, IBD, arteriovenous malformation, juvenile polyps, Peutz–Jeghers syndrome, familial adenomatous polyposis, solitary rectal ulcer syndrome, and trauma and child sexual abuse.

33–36. Answers:

33. I
34. A
35. M
36. J

Recurrent abdominal pain

Recurrent abdominal pain presenting with other features such as weight loss, growth and pubertal delay, or perianal problems such as tags, fissures or ulcers may indicate IBD. A strong family history may suggest diseases such as polyps, IBD, migraine and gastric ulcers. Persisting vomiting and cyclic vomiting should alert one to look for a cause such as a metabolic disorder or increased intracranial pressure. Dysphagia, haematemesis or rectal bleeding associated with abdominal pain should be taken seriously – an investigation to find the underlying cause is needed. Fever can be due to many bacterial, viral, immunological and idiopathic causes in patients with abdominal pain. Erythema nodosum with abdominal pain may indicate viral infection, IBD or TB. Diarrhoea or constipation in children with recurrent abdominal pain need a wider plan of investigation to find the cause. Arthritis may also be associated with abdominal pain.

Neurology

BOFs

1. The following are all characteristic features of hereditary motor sensory neuropathy type I except:

   A Vasomotor disturbances are common.
   B Sensory abnormalities are severe.
   C A high-stepping gait is common.
   D There is an onion bulb formation round nerve fibres.
   E There is extensive segmental demyelination of nerve fibres.

2. In Guillain–Barré syndrome, all of the following are true except:

   A It is characterized by progressive weakness.
   B Demyelination of peripheral nerves rarely occurs.
   C Facial nerves are often involved.
   D Deep tendon reflexes are lost early in most cases.
   E It may be associated with cardiac arrhythmia.

3. The characteristic features associated with Miller–Fisher syndrome include the following except:

   A Ataxia
   B Lower pyramidal tract signs
   C Ophthalmoplegia
   D Bulbar palsy
   E High CSF protein

4. What is the most useful test for myasthenia gravis in a 2-year-old girl?

   A Muscle biopsy
   B Nerve conduction study
   C Electromyography
   D Tensoline test
   E Acetylcholine receptor antibodies

5. In spinal muscular dystrophy (Werdnig–Hoffmann disease), one answer is correct from the following:

   A It is inherited in an autosomal dominant manner.
   B Patients can survive until their teens.
   C It is associated with a deletion of axon 7 of the *SMN* gene in over 95% of cases.
   D Pathology shows a loss of pyramidal tracts.
   E Serum creatine kinase is usually high.

6. The treatment of choice for benign rolandic epilepsy of childhood is:

   A Carbamazepine
   B Nothing
   C Sodium valproate
   D Prednisolone
   E Vigabatrin

7. The first drug of choice for absence epilepsy syndrome of childhood is:

   A Lamotrigine
   B Topiramate
   C Phenytoin
   D Sodium valproate
   E Carbamazepine

8. Common causes of nystagmus include the following except:

   A Neuroblastoma
   B Gaucher's disease
   C Congenital
   D Chiari malformations
   E Posterior fossa tumours

9. In moyamoya disease, which of the following is true:

   A It is progressive stenosis of large blood vessels at the base of the brain.
   B It is inherited as an X-linked recessive disorder.
   C Bleeding is a common manifestation.
   D Chorea may be a presenting feature.
   E Bilateral weakness is common.

10. The following are commonly associated with Sturge–Weber syndrome:

A Tramline appearance on skull x-ray
B Venous haemangiomas of the leptomeninges
C Glaucoma
D Mental retardation in more than one-third of patients
E Seizures usually occurring in the first month of life

11. The following are features of post-haemorrhagic hydrocephalus except:

A It commonly follows head trauma in older children.
B Neonatal IVH is the cause in premature babies.
C Ventricular dilation occurs very rapidly.
D A ventriculoperitoneal shunt is not indicated in most cases.
E It may be associated with ataxia.

12. The following are common manifestations of raised intracranial pressure in a 10-year-old child as a result of intracranial tumours except:

A Headaches
B Early-morning sickness
C Papilloedema is absent in half of affected children
D Large head
E Diplopia

13. The following changes are often associated with craniopharyngioma except:

A Dilated lateral ventricles
B Papilloedema
C Delayed growth
D Ipsilateral hemianopia
E Calcification of a tumour (less frequent)

14. Causes of vasogenic cerebral oedema include the following except:

A Meningitis
B Cerebral tumours
C Hypoxic–ischaemic encephalopathy cerebral infarct
D Inappropriate ADH secretion
E Encephalitis

15. **The following regarding febrile convulsions are true except:**

    A The recurrence rate is 30% after the first febrile convulsion.
    B In 15% of cases, they may be caused by meningitis.
    C They are usually familial.
    D Sodium valproate for 2 years is the treatment of choice.
    E 1–1.2% of children may develop epilepsy in adulthood.

16. **The following are all true about migraines in children except:**

    A More than 60% of headaches are unilateral.
    B A cranial MRI scan will help in diagnosis.
    C They are often familial.
    D An aura is not present in most cases.
    E Sumatriptan is not licensed for use in children under the age of 12 years.

17. **Lethargy, irritability and a sleepy child will suggest a diagnosis of encephalitis if the patient has:**

    A Seizures
    B Low serum sodium
    C Altered level of consciousness
    D Fixed neurological deficit
    E High serum white cell count

18. **Which of the following features is associated with temporal lobe epilepsy:**

    A Déjà vu
    B Auditory hallucinations
    C 3 Hz spike wave activity on EEG
    D Personality problems
    E Fumbling movements

19. **What is the most rare sign associated with subdural effusion in infants with suspicion of non-accidental injury?**

    A Seizures
    B Fever
    C Hemiplegia
    D Raised anterior fontanelle
    E Retinal haemorrhages

EMQs

20–24. For each of the following scenarios, select the most likely diagnosis from the list below:

20. A 7-year-old boy has a history of focal seizures at night. He will wake up and walk to parents' bedroom, drooling from his mouth on the left side, jerking the left side of his body, and is unable to talk. This never happens during the daytime, and he is doing well at school. His EEG shows central–temporal spikes.

21. A 7-month-old infant presents with a history of loss of consciousness on two occasions. This starts with him crying as if in pain, which is then followed by cessation of breathing and cyanosis with stiffening of the body before loss of consciousness. The EEG is normal, and there is no developmental delay.

22. A 13-year-old boy is diagnosed as having pendular nystagmus that becomes worse on looking to either side. He wears glasses to correct the vision of his right eye. His hair, eyelashes and eyebrows are blond. He is not clumsy and does not have a tremor.

23. A 2-day-old baby was born by elective LSCS for previous LSCS. He has proximal weakness and is hypotonic. There are no reflexes over the next 3 weeks, with marked symmetrical hypotonia. His chest is flattened laterally, with paradoxical respiration. There is abnormal movement of his tongue, and he is no longer able to suck. He is very alert and starts to smile. A cranial MRI is normal, and an EMG shows polyphasic motor unit potentials with increased duration.

24. A 12-year-old girl has a history of frequent falls and has difficulty in running. She has pes cavus with symmetrical atrophy of the peroneal muscles. The ankle reflexes are lost, with mild sensory loss in the lower limbs only. A nerve conduction study shows marked delay in enervation.

Options

A Ataxia telangiectasia
B Motor sensory neuropathy type I
C Hypoxic–ischaemic encephalopathy
D Spastic quadriplegia
E Temporal lobe epilepsy
F Breath-holding attack
G Generalized tonic clonic seizure disorder
H Spinal muscle atrophy
I Benign rolandic epilepsy of childhood
J Dancing eye syndrome
K Refsum's disease
L Oculocutaneous albinism
M Friedreich's ataxia
N Sciatic nerve palsy
O Myasthenia gravis
P Mitochondrial cytopathy

25–28. For each of the following scenarios, select the investigation most likely to give a definite diagnosis from the list below:

25. A 2-year-old child with left eye glaucoma is developmentally delayed and has multiple seizure types. His renal scan shows small cortical cystic lesions. The EEG shows hypsarrhythmia. He is on vigabatrin and topiramate.

26. A 7-day-old baby girl has been diagnosed with Horner's syndrome. She is unable to move her right arm. Delivery was difficult, with shoulder dystocia and required forceps. No fractures are noted, and a cranial CT scan is reported as normal.

27. An 11-year-old boy has a history of blurred vision in both eyes, the left more than the right, and double vision when looking to either side. Fundus examination shows papilloedema more on the left. A cranial MRI is normal as in a VEP. A DNA study for Farber's disease is normal.

28. A 4-year-old girl has a history of clumsiness and frequently falls over. Her foot arch is very high, with reduced reflexes at her ankles. Her bladder and bowel control are good. She finds it difficult to rise from a sitting to a standing position and has to use her arms to raise her body. Peroneal nerve conduction and cranial MRI are normal. Creatinine kinase is 250 mmol/l.

Options
A Nerve conduction study
B Cranial MRI
C Electrical retinography
D Cranial CT
E Lumbar puncture for measuring pressure
F Lumbar puncture for lactate and CSF oligoclonal bands
G Skin biopsy
H Muscle biopsy
I Serum creatinine kinase
J Sleep study EEG
K Serum organic acids
L Chromosome study
M DMSA scan
N Wood's light test

29–33. For each of the following case scenarios, select the most likely diagnosis from the list below:

29. A 10-year-old girl walks with flexion hips and flexion knees and falls forward. Her Achilles tendon is very tight and all of her reflexes are brisk. She attends normal school, but her expressive language is delayed. A cranial MRI scan shows generalized cortical atrophy with mild dilated ventricles.

30. A 15-year-old girl is diagnosed with epilepsy and treated with carbamazepine and sodium valproate. Most of her seizures occur on the left side, with hallucinations and fumbling with her clothes. She always runs to her mother before each attack. At the age of 10 months, she had a prolonged febrile convulsion for an hour and a half. The MRI scan shows left hippocampal sclerosis.

31. A 5-year-old girl has a history of irritability and drowsiness, a temperature of 38°C, and equally reactive pupils. She is alert, with normal capillary refill time. Her LP shows 10 lymphocytes only. Her CSF glucose is 3 mmol/l and serum glucose 5 mmol/l. CSF protein is 40 mg and no organisms are seen. An EEG shows slow background activity.

32. A 13-year-old girl has been sleeping excessively and has a headache. Her cranial CT shows supracellular calcification. Her weight is on the 90th centile; she is sleepy and has said many times that she has hit the side of her head when coming close to corners. She is not enjoying school and has been bullied because of her weight. Both parents are unemployed and heavy smokers. A cousin died from cystic fibrosis at the age of 10 years with a brain tumour.

33. A child is brought to Casualty with saliva drooling from the right corner of his mouth. He cannot talk properly but can swallow drinks. He attended his friend's birthday party 2 days ago and said he drank one glass of wine. There is drooping of his face on the right side, and is unable to close his right eye. There is a rash around his right ear that looks crusty and pink. He says that his ear has hurt him for the last 2 days. There is no hearing loss, and he has been fully vaccinated. He had chickenpox at the age of 6 years and suffers from cold sores. A full blood count and film show raised lymphocytes only. The cranial MRI is reported as normal.

Options

A   Benign increased intracranial pressure
B   Third-nerve palsy
C   Prolonged febrile convulsions
D   Periventricular calcification
E   Duchenne muscular dystrophy
F   Spastic diplegic cerebral palsy
G   Shoulder dystocia
H   Klumpke's paralysis
I   McCune–Albright syndrome
J   Sacular aneurysm
K   Status epilepticus
L   Encephalitis
M   Hyperglycinaemia and encephalopathy
N   Craniopharyngioma
O   Subarachnoid haemorrhage
P   Ramsay Hunt syndrome
Q   Bell's palsy
R   Kayser–Fleischer ring
S   Glaucoma
T   Vein of Galen malformation
U   Guillain–Barré syndrome
V   Temporal lobe epilepsy

Answers for Neurology

1. Answer: B

Hereditary motor sensory neuropathy

This is a group of genetic neuropathies with an incidence of 10 per 100 000 of the population. The commonest is HMSN type 1: Charcot–Marie–Tooth disease. It is autosomal dominant, with peroneal atrophy. In many cases, the abnormal gene is on chromosome 17. The initial symptoms are either foot deformities or gait disturbances beginning in the 2nd decade and sometimes in early infancy. Pes cavus is typical, and hammertoes may be present. All of these weaknesses are caused by weakness of the intrinsic foot muscles. Gait is described as a neuropathic gait, with the feet being lifted up and dropped on the floor, and the child is described as clumsy. Initially, examination will show atrophy of the peroneal muscles, pes cavus and reduced reflexes of the Achilles tendon. The disease is progressive and leads to more muscle weakness that may affect the proximal and distal muscles, foot drop and cramps with normal sensation. In adults, peripheral nerves are enlarged, which is caused by repeated episodes of demyelination and remyelination. Nerve conduction studies are diagnostic, along with a muscle biopsy in cases with a normal nerve conduction study. There is no specific treatment, but supportive care with proper foot care should be given.

Other types of HMSN include types II, III (Déjerine–Sottas disease) and IV (Refsum's disease).

2. Answer: B

Guillain–Barré syndrome

The initial symptoms are weakness and paraesthesia in the distal portion of the limbs. Facial weakness can also occur in 15% of cases. There is continuous or relapsing motor and sensory dysfunction in more than one limb over at least 2 months, areflexia or hyporeflexia that usually affects all four limbs. There is usually no family history, just pure sensory neuropathy or abnormal storage material in the nerves. The CSF is high in protein, with low motor nerve conduction velocity and features of demyelination on nerve biopsy. Intravenous immunoglobulin proves to be effective if given early. Steroids are another option.

3. Answer: D

Miller–Fisher syndrome

This is characterized by ataxia, ophthalmoplegia and areflexia. It is a variant of Guillian–Barré syndrome. Half of the patients will have had a viral illness 10–15 days before it started. A common ocular manifestation is paralysis of the vertical gaze; the upward gaze is more severely affected. The horizontal gaze is not affected. Ataxia is more common in the limbs than the trunk, with bilateral or unilateral facial weakness. Recovery occurs within 2–4 weeks. CSF protein is high. The outcome in untreated patients is excellent. Steroids, IVIG and plasmapheresis have been tried, without much benefit.

4. Answer: D

Myasthenia gravis

The weakness usually improves after intravenous administration of edrophonium chloride. A group of patients will not show much improvement with an intravenous infusion, but will improve with an intramuscular infusion, especially young children with no venous access. The test should be done in hospital with a PICU bed booked beforehand. About 70% patients, adults or children, with acquired generalized myasthenia and 54% with ocular myasthenia have serum antibodies that bind human acetylcholine receptor (AChR). Antibodies may be low at the beginning of the illness but will elevate later, and 10% of cases may show other types of autoantibodies on tissue culture. AChR-binding antibodies may increase in patients with systemic lupus erythematosus, inflammatory neuropathy or amyotrophic lateral sclerosis, in rheumatoid arthritis patients taking D-penicillamine, in patients with thymoma without myasthenia gravis and in normal relatives of patients with myasthenia gravis. False-positive results occur in patients who have had surgery within the last 48 hours under general anaesthesia. In electromyography repetitive nerve stimulation (RNS), the amplitude of the compound muscle action potential (CMAP) elicited by repetitive nerve stimulation is normal or only slightly reduced in patients without myasthenia gravis. Single-fibre EMG is positive in newly all cases of myasthenia gravis, and will show increased jitters in some muscles. It is also the most sensitive clinical test of neuromuscular transmission.

5. Answer: C

Central hypotonia

All hypotonic babies and infants look much the same, regardless of the cause, when lying supine. The thighs are fully abducted (froglike position), and the arms lie in a flaccid position beside the head with marked head lag when they are lifted up by the hands. There are many causes of hypotonia in newborn babies, including cerebral hypotonia-like chromosomal disorders, cerebral malformation, paroxysmal disorders, Lowe's syndrome, metabolic defects, spinal cord disorders, spinal muscular atrophies, transient neonatal myasthenia gravis, congenital muscular dystrophies and polyneuropathies. Cerebral hypotonia, is usually associated with other anomalies of brain function, dysmorphic features, fisting of hands, malformation of other organs, normal or brisk tendon reflexes, scissoring on vertebral suspension and movement through postural reflexes. Motor unit disorders are characterized by absent or depressed tendon reflexes, failure of movement on postural reflexes, fasciculation and muscle atrophy, with no abnormalities of other organs. There are many causes, but transient hypotonia does exist. Looking for a cause should be linked to clinical examination findings. Family history as well as pregnancy details are helpful in diagnosis.

6. Answer: B

Benign rolandic epilepsy of childhood

This is characterized by seizures at night where the child goes to sleep and the parents hear noises, or the child comes to the parents with mouth open and unable to talk. Most of the time, the child feels a tingling in their mouth that is followed by seizures, which can be focal. About 10% of seizures may occur during the daytime. A sleep EEG will show centrotemporal spikes, but the awake EEG will be normal. Drugs can be used if seizures become multiple or occur during daytime. Using carbamazepine can cause some problems in children. Clobazam is good if given just once a day at night.

7. Answer: D

AEDs for absence epilepsy syndrome

Childhood absence epilepsy syndrome is the most common primary generalized epilepsy in children between the ages of 3 and 9 years. It is characterized by brief absences or staring with eye flickering, sometimes followed by mouth movement or swallowing. It can be frequent, with no cause being found. It is characterized by polyspike waves at 3 Hz. Sodium valproate is a good choice for girls under 10 years and lamotrigine for those over 10 years. Boys can have sodium valproate. Ethosuximide is also effective as single or add-on therapy. New drugs such as topiramate and levetiracetam have not yet proven superior to others, but can be tried if others fail. Prognosis is good in the majority of children.

8. Answer: B

Nystagmus

Physiological nystagmus that is congenital and associated with blindness can be familial or idiopathic. Spasmus nutans is a form of nystagmus and can be due to an optic nerve tumour or idiopathic in origin. Pendular nystagmus can be due to brainstem tumours, ictal nystagmus, multiple sclerosis or oculopalatal syndrome. Horizontal pendular jerking can be due to drugs or vestibular or vertical nystagmus.

9. Answer: C

Moyamoya disease

This is a slowly progressive disease due to the occlusion of the internal carotid arteries and sometimes the basilar artery. Following this, multiple anastomoses will appear between the internal and external carotid arteries. Headaches can be the first sign, followed by abrupt hemiplegia. Recovery will follow, but this is usually followed by another attack of hemiparesis involving the face and eyes and sometimes with chorea affecting one side of the face or limbs. Transient ischaemic attacks are a manifestation of this disease. A CT scan may show an infarction, but MRA or arteriography will be diagnostic. Recanalization can be effective, as can verapamil.

10. Answer: C

Sturge–Weber syndrome

Seizures occur in up to 90% of these cases and are usually focal and occur in the first year of life. Mental retardation is common, and hemiplegia of the contralateral side occurs in half of patients. Seizures are often difficult to treat, so children will be considered for hemispherectomy.

11. Answer: C

Post-haemorrhagic hydrocephalus

This occurs more with grade III or IV of IVH which is due to plugging of the arachnoid villi and impaired absorption of CSF. Ventricular dilation can occur without an increase in the size of the head by initial pressure on brain tissue. Hydrocephalus may arrest in at least one-third to two-thirds of cases, or may progress to a severe form. A ventriculoperitoneal shunt cannot be performed until the blood clot has been absorbed; otherwise there is a risk of blockage, and the risk of infection will increase. Treatment using ventricular washout during the acute phase is still in its early stages, and results are yet to be seen.

12. Answer: D

Raised intracranial pressure

Common symptoms in infants are bulging fontanelles, failure to thrive, a large head, setting sun sign and a shrill cry. In older children, the symptoms are diplopia, headaches, mental changes, nausea and vomiting, and papilloedema.

13. Answer: A

Intracranial lesions associated with calcification

These include oligodendroglioma (50%), astrocytoma (20%), glioma (10%), meningioma (15%), metastases and craniopharyngioma (90% children, 40% adults) and chordoma (50%). Others include pituitary adenoma, pinealoma, lipoma, harmatoma, teratoma, and dermoid, epidermoid and choroid plexus papilloma.

14. Answer: C

Vasogenic cerebral oedema

Cerebral oedema may follow many conditions, including Reye's syndrome, benign intracranial hypertension, excess fluid infusion in a dehydrated/ hypernatraemic patient and acute hepatic failure. It can also (rarely) be associated with diabetic ketoacidosis if fluid is given rapidly at high altitude (above 3500–4000 metres).

Cerebral oedema can take the following forms. The vasogenic form is caused by excess protein-rich fluid leaking into the extracellular space through damaged capillaries, and it particularly affects the white matter. Treatment with steroids can be effective. Cytotoxic oedema represents intracellular damage within the neurones and glia. Interstitial oedema usually follows leakage of CSF into the extracellular space (e.g. in non-communicating hydrocephalus).

15. Answer: D

Febrile convulsions

Fever is one of the commonest causes of convulsions in infants and children under 5 years of age and sometimes up to 7 years. Febrile convulsions are usually familial, with the mode of inheritance being autosomal dominant in certain families. In some families, genetic markers have been identified. Febrile convulsions usually follow a viral infection, but also occur in 15% of children presenting with meningitis under the age of 5 years. Urinary tract and upper respiratory tract infections are among the commonest causes. Children presenting for the first time with febrile convulsions should be admitted and the focus of infection found in all cases. Parents are usually terrified – so they should be provided with written information and told when to ask for help. There is no need to give any antiepileptic drugs, but rectal diazepam can be given for those with prolonged febrile convulsions or having had recurrent longer attacks for more than 5 minutes. No EEG or cranial CT is required. The normal prevalence of epilepsy in the childhood population is 1–1.2%.

16. Answer: B

Migraine

Headaches are one of the commonest reasons for referrals to the neurology clinic. They can be chronic and non-progressive, in which case no urgent investigation is needed and treatment can be started with simple analgesia and then proceed to use β-blockers and antiepileptics. Sometimes a multidisciplinary team approach is good. The acute headache over a short period with neurological deficit needs urgent attention, and investigations should be performed immediately. Migraine is an acute headache, but usually happens once a week or month and is usually associated with a strong family history. More than 50% of cases are not unilateral headaches, and the classical picture of a migraine does not always accompany the attack. History of pain in the stomach, blurred vision and pain in the throat are warning signs. A headache will follow, and may be associated with photophobia, blurred vision and vomiting in many cases. The headache may last from 1 hour up to 2–3 days. Sleeping in a dark, quiet room with analgesia will help a lot. Triptans are not licensed for use in children, but various studies have proven them to be as effective as in adults.

17. Answer: E

Encephalitis

This can present at any age, and the presentation varies. Viral infections are the main cause of encephalitis, but metabolic disorders can also be responsible. In viral encephalitis, the presentation can be as acute onset of fever, headache, lethargy, nausea and vomiting. Irritability, off feeding, seizures and lethargy in infants is another presentation. Seizures are common, with some neurological deficit, especially with herpes simplex encephalitis. Fluctuations of symptoms are common, with bizarre behaviour, sleepiness and drowsiness for 10–15 minutes then back to normal. The symptoms can get worse, and the child will lapse into a coma and require ventilatory support. The blood tests are usually normal, and a lumbar puncture is not specific, with few white cells, red cells, normal or low glucose, and normal protein. PCR for HSV and other viruses is now helpful to rule these out. An EEG will show focal abnormalities and temporal lobe discharges as in HSV encephalitis. Enhanced CT may show the focal infected area, and an MRI is more specific. Supportive treatment, antivirals, antibiotics and control of seizures are what the patient needs. Mortality and morbidity with HSV encephalitis is high, but is less with other viruses.

18. Answer: C

Temporal lobe epilepsy

This is the most common cause of complex partial seizures. Most cases are symptomatic, although sometimes there is difficulty in demonstrating a lesion that is epileptogenic in nature. The condition in children is similar to that in adults in terms of its origin, and its onset is with behaviour arrest and staring. Automatism is mainly in the form of lip-smacking, licking, chewing or swallowing in younger children, while older children may exhibit gesturing automatisms such as fingering or fumbling with clothes. Tonic posturing and head rotation are more common in children under the age of 2 years. The seizure may last 1–2 minutes, and is then followed by a period of confusion and tiredness. Complex seizures of temporal lobe origin are usually preceded by auras with hallucination or illusions. In young children, epigastric pain is the commonest aura, while in younger ones head posturing or deviation may be an indication of aura. Mesial temporal lobe sclerosis is common in older children and is associated with atrophy and gliosis of the hippocampus and often the amygdala. A history of prolonged febrile seizures is found in approximately 40–50% of patients with hippocampal sclerosis. Cortical dysplasia localized to the temporal lobe can lead to complex partial seizures and temporal lobe epilepsy. MRI is very good in picking up abnormalities affecting the temporal lobe. The EEG can be normal, but repeated studies are very important; and sometimes videotelemetry may be needed if surgical evaluation is required. Carbamazepine, oyxcarbazepine, topiramate, lamotrigine and levetiracetam are all effective in the treatment of complex partial seizures.

19. Answer: B

Subdural effusion in infants

This usually follows head trauma, although in some cases there is no clear history of trauma. There is a collection bilaterally in 85% of cases, and the pathophysiology of the subdural haematoma is not yet fully understood. It occurs mainly in infants between the age of 2 and 9 months. The head is enlarged, the anterior fontanelle is tense or bulging, and the eyes may show sun-setting signs. Retinal and preretinal haemorrhage presents in half of the cases and is strongly suggestive of a non-accidental injury. Focal neurological deficits are uncommon, and hemiparesis may occur. Seizures may also occur. A CT will show enlargement of the pericerebral spaces, with compressed ventricles and displaced sulci. Parenchymal lesions in the form of haemorrhages or multiple areas of oedematous density are often present. Evacuation of the collection to relieve the pressure on the brain can be performed in a specialist centre, and can be repeated. If the child develops hydrocephalus, a VP shunt should be considered.

20–24. Answers:

20. I: Benign rolandic epilepsy of childhood usually starts between 7 and 13 years of age, but can occur in younger children as well. Ten percent usually occur during daytime. No neuroimaging is required, even if the EEG is focal and seizures are focal. If the seizures occur during the daytime or are more frequent, carbamazepine, clobazam or sodium valproate will help. Very rarely, it will evolve to chronic-type epilepsy.

21. F: Breath-holding attacks occur in children as young as 3 months. The child will stop breathing and have no inspiratory phase. He/she will just breathe out but not in, and after a couple of minutes will turn blue, fall on the ground and may have seizures. This is an anoxic reflux seizure, which does not need any further testing. The best way to find out is to ask the parents to video it.

22. L: There are many types of oculocutaneous albinism due to partial or complete failure of production of melanin in the skin, eyes and hair. It is characterized by absence of tyrosinase activity and usually presents as photophobia, nystagmus, defective visual acuity, white hair and white skin.

23. H: In newborns, spinal muscular atrophy presents as hypotonia. It can be recognized in utero by decreased fetal movements. The majority of affected infants breathe adequately at birth and appear very alert, as facial features are preserved very well although the rest of the body is weak. Eye movement is normal. Paradoxical respiration will develop because of paralysis of the intercostal muscles, with impaired diaphragm movement. It is usually not associated with arthrogryposis. Spinal muscular atrophy is a progressive disease, and infants will start to lose their gag reflex, with difficulty in feeding, and they usually die from a chest infection or aspiration. CK is usually normal. EMG will show fibrillation and fasciculations at rest and increased mean amplitudes of motor unit potentials. A muscle biopsy will establish the diagnosis.

24. B: See answer to Question 1.

25–28. Answers:

25. B: Aicardi's syndrome – Look for evidence of callosal agenesis, cystic lesions, olivopontine abnormalities and dilated ventricles. It is also characterized by ocular abnormalities, dysmorphic facies, cleft lip, cleft palate, seizures, epilepsy, infantile spasms, mental retardation, hemivertebrae, fused vertebrae, rib abnormalities, scoliosis, chorioretinal lacunae, pathognomonic lesions and retinal colobomata.

26. A: Klumpke's palsy results in deficits at levels C8 and T1, although many clinicians agree that pure C8–T1 injuries do not occur in infants and may be indicative of spinal cord injury (SCI). An infant with a nerve injury to the lower plexus (C8–T1) holds the arm supinated with the elbow bent and the wrist extended. Reflexes are typically absent in the affected limb and should be evaluated. This examination is particularly important in distinguishing BPP from hemiparesis. Reflexes do not typically return except in the mildest injuries. The most common associated injuries (not causative) include clavicular and humeral fractures, torticollis cephalohaematoma, facial nerve palsy and diaphragmatic paralysis.

27. C, E: Benign increased intracranial pressure. This most commonly affects teenagers, particularly those who are overweight. The common sign is papilloedema, although this is absent in some cases. Occasionally, patients may present with abducens or other cranial nerve palsies. Symptoms include severe headaches, visual disturbances (diplopia), nausea/vomiting and pulsatile tinnitus. Risk factors include female gender, overweight, excess *or* deficiency of vitamin A, and some medications. Diagnosis is by exclusion of any intracranial tumors or masses. A CT will help to exclude any mass effect, and LP will confirm the diagnosis.

The aim is to reduce the pressure: repeated LP can produce a reduction of 25%, which most cannot tolerate; acetazolamide can also be useful. Consider repeating blood gas determination. Corticosteroids can also be used, and a lumboperitoneal shunt can be performed in extreme cases. It is important to save the child's vision.

28. H: The most common genetic myopathies are Duchenne and Becker muscular dystrophies, resulting from a genetic defect on the X chromosome. These need to be distinguished from autoimmune disorders (e.g. myasthenia gravis, scleroderma and thyroiditis), endocrine disorders (e.g. Cushing's syndrome, hypothyroidism, hyperthyroidism and Addison's disease), exposure to toxins (e.g. herbicides, insecticides and flame-retardant chemicals), infection (e.g. HIV, Lyme disease and trichinosis), vitamin D deficiency, vitamin E or A toxicity, medication (e.g. some antihistamines and long-term corticosteroid use) and metabolic disorders (e.g. glycogen and lipid storage diseases).

29–33. Answers:

29. F: Spastic diplegic cerebral palsy is characterized by upper motor neurone findings in the legs and more so than the arms, a scissoring gait pattern with hips flexed and adducted, knees flexed with valgus and ankles in equinus (resulting in toe-walking), learning disabilities, and seizures (less commonly than in spastic hemiplegia).

30. V: Temporal lobe epilepsy (see answer to Question 18).

31. L: Encephalitis (see answer to Question 17).

32. N: Craniopharyngioma is characterized by headaches that are slow and progressive, dull, continuous, and positional. On presentation, 40% of patients will have symptoms of hypothyroidism (e.g. weight gain, fatigue, cold intolerance and constipation). Almost 25% have associated signs and symptoms of adrenal failure (e.g. orthostatic hypotension, hypoglycaemia, hyperkalaemia, cardiac arrhythmias, lethargy, confusion, anorexia, and nausea and vomiting) and 20% have diabetes insipidus (e.g. excessive fluid intake and urination). Most young patients present with growth failure and delayed puberty. Optic pathway dysfunction on presentation is noted in 40–70% of patients. Children rarely become aware of visual problems (only 20–30%) and often present after almost complete visual damage has taken place. Thalamus and frontal lobes present with corresponding endocrine, autonomic and behavioural problems (e.g. hyperphagia and obesity, psychomotor retardation, emotional immaturity, apathy, short-term memory deficits, and incontinence). Short stature is present in 23–45% and obesity in 11–18%.

33. Q: Bell's palsy can be congenital, post herpes simplex infection, as part of Ramsey Hunt syndrome, due to HIV infections, or as a result of other causes, including facial and surgical wounds, blunt force trauma, temporal bone fractures, brainstem injuries, acoustic neuromas, cysts and tumours that result in facial palsy. Diabetes and thyroid conditions are also associated with facial palsy. Lupus, Sjögren's syndrome and congenital defects can, infrequently, cause facial paralysis.

Haematology and Oncology

BOFs

1. The following are true about aplastic anaemia except:

   A It is related to defective DNA repair.
   B There is an increased risk of acute myeloplastic leukaemia in patients with aplastic anaemia.
   C It is not associated with skin abnormalities.
   D Short stature is a common feature.
   E Thrombocytopenia is the initial change.

2. Which of the following is a feature of Diamond–Blackfan anaemia (DBA)?

   A It is inherited in an autosomal dominant manner.
   B The bone marrow is acellular with an increase in erythroid pre-cursors.
   C A cleft or high-arched palate is not very common.
   D An absent radius is associated with DBA.
   E Anaemia can be macrocytic or normocytic.

3. The following conditions are associated with the development of myeloid dysplasia in children except:

   A Neurofibromatosis type 1
   B Down's syndrome
   C Fanconi's anaemia
   D Previous radiation therapy
   E Idiopathic thrombocytopenic purpura

4. The following statements are true except:

   A Haem iron is taken up directly by specialized receptors in the mucosal membrane.
   B The absorption of non-haem iron is reduced by the absence of haem iron.
   C Apotransferrin is a mucosal cell transporter for iron and is secreted by the intestinal mucosa.
   D Transferrin is increased when liver-stored iron is low.
   E Ferritin is a water-soluble protein whose iron stores are relatively easily available for iron metabolism.

5. As the level of iron is reduced in the body, all of the following are reduced except:

   A Serum ferritin
   B Red blood cell volume
   C Red cell protoporphyrins
   D Haemosiderin
   E Marrow sideroblast percentages

6. The 3 mg/kg/day of iron is provided to a baby of 6 kg in weight by prescribing:

   A 15 mg ferrous sulfate
   B 54 mg ferrous fumarate
   C 9 mg ferrous succinate
   D 26 mg ferrous gluconate
   E 17 mg ferrous glycine sulfate

7. One of the following is a cause of megaloblastic anaemia:

   A Pernicious anaemia
   B Ileal resection
   C Fish tapeworm
   D Hereditary orotic aciduria
   E Gastro-oesophagitis

8. The following is true about erythropoesis after birth:

   A In the first week of life, the erythropoietin level will reach zero.
   B Haemoglobin production will start to increase after the second week of life until 12 weeks of age.
   C Red cell survival during the first 12 weeks will not change.
   D Bone marrow erythroid activity will increase between 3 and 4 weeks of age.
   E In hypoxic or anaemic neonates, erythropoietin levels are high in the first few weeks of life.

9. The following are causes of haemolysis in the first 6 weeks of life except:

   A Bacterial sepsis
   B Angiopathic haemolytic anaemia due to cavernous haemangioma
   C Sickle cell anaemia
   D Hereditary spherocytosis
   E Pyruvate kinase deficiency in red cells

10. **All of the following factors can contribute to the pathophysiology of anaemia of prematurity except:**

   A Frequent blood sampling
   B Neonatal reticulocytosis
   C Reduced lifespan of neonatal erythrocytes
   D Reduced tissue oxygen availability
   E Nutritional deficiencies

11. **The following drugs may cause autoimmune haemolytic anaemia except:**

   A Methyldopa
   B High doses of penicillin
   C Quinidine
   D Ibuprofen
   E α-Aminobenzoic acid

12. **The following are indications for the use of irradiated blood in neonates and paediatric patients except:**

   A Low birthweight of 1200 g
   B Infants undergoing exchange transfusion for Rh haemolytic diseases
   C HIV infection
   D Children with sickle cell anaemia
   E Known cellular immune-deficient patients

13. **Indications for using fresh frozen plasma include:**

   A Severe liver diseases
   B Disseminated intravascular coagulation
   C Massive transfusion
   D Treatment of haemophilia
   E Isolated congenital coagulation factor deficiency

14. **The following are vitamin K-dependent coagulation factors except:**

   A Protein C
   B Factor VII
   C Factor XII
   D Factor IX
   E Factor II (prothrombin)

15. The following are poor prognostic features of acute lymphoblastic leukaemia except:

   A Age less than 1 year
   B WCC $>100 \times 10^9$/l
   C Chromosome count >50
   D DNA index <1.16
   E M2 and M3 marrow

16. The characteristic features of L1 ALL according to the French–American–British (FAB) classification include all of the following except:

   A Cytoplasmic vacuolation is variable.
   B One or more nucleoli are prominent.
   C The cytoplasm is scanty.
   D Basophilia of the cytoplasm is slight or moderate.
   E The nuclear chromatin is homogenous.

EMQs

17–20. For each of the following scenarios choose the appropriate diagnosis from the list below:

   17. A 3-year-old boy presents with a history of increasing pallor, bruises and some petechial rashes. His full blood count shows pancytopenia with no other physical abnormalities. His grandfather died of leukaemia. The bone marrow shows erythroid hyperplasia. Chromosomal breakage using diepoxybutane shows no evidence of a DNA repair problem.

   18. A 15-month-old girl presents with a history of failure to thrive. She is below the 3rd centile for her weight and height, although she was born above the 25th centile. Her full blood count shows neutropenia and thrombocytopenia, and she is anaemic. No blast cells are seen on the blood film, and the bone marrow shows moderate erythroid hypoplasia. She has a malabsorption problem. Chromosomal breakage using diepoxybutane shows no increase in breakage.

   19. A 4-year-old boy presents with an increasing history of pallor and nosebleeds almost once a day for the last 3 days. He is diagnosed with a chronic condition associated with skin hyperkeratosis, dental decay, early loss of teeth, loss of hair and hyperhidrosis of the palms and soles. There is no increase in chromosomal breakage using diepoxybutane.

   20. A girl is born to a healthy mother after an event-free pregnancy. The radius is absent, but the thumb is preserved. Her platelet count is low.

Options

A Acute lymphoblastic leukaemia
B Fanconi's anaemia
C Shwachman–Diamond syndrome
D Acquired aplastic anaemia
E TAR syndrome
F Amegakaryocytic thrombocytopenia syndrome
G Dyskeratosis congenita
H Kostmann's syndrome
I Seckel's syndrome

21–24. Choose from the following scenarios the most appropriate diagnosis from the list below:

21. A 1-month-old infant boy presents with a change in the colour of his urine. He was born at term without any antenatal problems. He required facial oxygen but recovered quickly. Examination reveals a large mass on the right side of his abdomen. The urine shows macro- and microscopic haematuria. The platelet count is low, but haemoglobin is 12.3 g/dl. Abdominal ultrasound shows an enlarged right kidney with increased echogenicity.

22. A 2-month-old child presents to Casualty with a history of bleeding after a circumcision performed by the local doctor. He is the first child in his family, his mother is healthy and his mother said no other member of the family has a similar condition. He receives treatment, and the bleeding stops. The prothrombin time is prolonged. The partial thromboplastin time is also prolonged, with a normal thrombin time and bleeding time.

23. A 13-year-old boy presents with a history of tiredness, constipation and not feeling well. In the last few days, he has noticed a swelling of his neck and shortness of breath when he lies down. The full blood count shows mild anaemia with a slight increase in ALT, and the total bilirubin is 30 mmol/l. The chest X-ray shows a mediastinal mass extending to the neck. The liver is enlarged, with increased echogenicity, like the kidneys. A biopsy from the mass in the neck shows large cells and CD1–CD8 T-cell markers with positive CD10 in precursor B cells.

24. A 2-year-old girl presents with bruises on her legs and looks pale. She has been seen twice before for similar problems, with her mother being assured nothing was wrong. Examination shows a few petechial rashes on her legs and a few bruises on her shins and forehead. She looks tired and fragile. The full blood count shows a high white cell count, thrombocytopenia and a haemoglobin of 9.1 g/dl. A haematologist looks at the film and reports it as normal, but asks to perform a bone marrow biopsy, which shows over 40% lymphoblasts, with DNA testing showing chromosomal aberrations resulting in leukaemic fusion genes and fusion mRNA.

Options

A Hodgkin's lymphoma
B Acute myeloid leukaemia (AML)
C Lymphoblastic non-Hodgkin's lymphoma (NHL)
D Right renal vein thrombosis (RVT)
E Right iliac vein thrombosis
F Acute lymphoblastic leukaemia (ALL)
G Thyroid carcinoma
H Haemophilia type A
I Haemophilia
J T-cell lymphoma
K Burkitt's NHL
L Christmas disease
M Von Willebrand's disease
N Idiopathic thrombocytic purpura

25–28. For the following scenarios, choose the most appropriate investigation(s) of lymphocytic disorders from the list below:

25. A 6-month-old infant presents a second time with lobar pneumonia affecting the right upper lobe (on the previous occasion, the left lower lobe had been affected). There has been marked lymphopenia on two occasions. The chest X-ray also shows abnormal metaphysical dysplasia of costochondral junctions of all the ribs. IgE, IgM and IgG are high, with a positive Coombs' test and a low platelet count. A diagnosis is made, and a bone marrow transplantation is performed with excellent results.

26. A 9-month-old boy presents with skin rashes. He has had clobetasol propionate cream on two occasions; this helped to clear up the condition, only for it to recur after 3 weeks. The eczema is spreading on his face and legs. He is admitted to the ward with possible septicaemia due to infected eczema. His WCC is 14×10^9, platelets 30×10^9/l and Hb 12 g/dl.

27. A 2-year-old boy presents with a swollen, red, tender and hot left knee. A diagnosis of septic arthritis is made and staphylococci isolated. He is treated, but 2 months later presents with right upper lobe pneumonia and septicaemia. There is a very low number of B cells in the peripheral venous blood.

28. A 1-month-old baby is admitted with a chest infection. He has not yet gained back his birthweight and looks skinny. There is an enlarged spleen of 2 cm, with no liver enlargement. There are erythematous skin rashes all over his body. His blood culture grows streptococcal pneumonia, and he is treated with antibiotics for 5 days. His chest X-ray looks patchy and granular, and he continues to need oxygen after 7 days of admission. The cervical lymph nodes become enlarged, and his Heaf test is grade 2. Gastric aspirate and bronchoveolar lavage do not show any evidence of mycobacteria.

Options
A Calcium level
B Antibody titres for polio and measles
C IgG subclass
D IgG level
E Adenosine deaminase enzyme level
F CD4/CD8 ratio
G PCR for HIV genomic RNA
H IgA, IgM and IgE
I DNA radiation of cells
J Nitro blue test
K *WASP* gene

Answers for Haematology and Oncology

1. Answer: C

Aplastic anaemia

This is autosomal recessive and is characterized by hyperpigmented skin anomalies, which is the commonest anomaly. There are also upper limb abnormalities, hypogonadal and genitalia abnormalities, skeletal anomalies of head, neck and spine, epicanthal and eyelid anomalies, renal anomalies (e.g. horeshoe, pelvic or ectopic kidneys), deafness, external ear anomalies, and hip, foot and leg anomalies. The haematological features include thrombocytopenia, which is first to develop and is followed by agranulocytopenia and anaemia. Red cells are macrocytic, there is increased fetal haemoglobin, and bone marrow will show erythroid hyperplasia and sometimes dyserythropoiesis or megaloblastic-appearing cells. As the disease progresses, the marrow becomes hypocellular and fatty.

2. Answer: B

Diamond–Blackfan anaemia

This is sporadic in about 80 % of cases, but some families inherit this condition as AR, X-linked or AD. The anaemia can start in the neonatal period in 25 % of patients, but recognizing DBA may be later in life or early if there is a family history. In 50 % of patients, there are other anomalies – craniofacial anomalies being the most common, for example hyperthelorism, flat nasal bridge, and cleft or high-arched palate. There are thumb abnormalities in 10–20 %, ranging from a flat thenar eminence to an absent radius. In some cases, there is deafness or learning difficulties. They usually present at 2–3 months of age. The anaemia is associated with reticulocytopenia. The white cell count and platelets are normal or raised. There is a reduction in erythroid precursors in the bone marrow, with normal myeloid and megakaryocytic differentiation. Raised levels of erythrocyte adenosine deaminase in red cells have been described in a high proportion of patients, but this is not diagnostic, as it is high in other conditions (e.g. leukaemia and myelodysplastic syndromes). Steroids remain the mainstay of treatment. Between 40 and 50 % of patients will still need regular transfusions. Cyclosporine, erythropoietin and IV immunoglobulin are other treatment modalities. Bone marrow transplantation is very successful in 60–70 % of patients and can be curative.

3. Answer: E

Myeloid dysplasia

Other conditions associated with myeloid dysplasia include trisomy 18, Kostmann's syndrome, Diamond–Blackfan anaemia, Shwachman–Diamond syndrome, familial myeloid dysplasia, and aplastic anaemia due to immuno-suppressive therapy or cytotoxic therapy. Pallor is common. Bacterial infections can be due to neutropenia or defective neutrophil function. Lymph node enlargement is unusual, with spleen and liver enlargement not being universal. Characteristic skin rashes such as Langerhan's cell histiocytosis may occur on the face or trunk. The blasts are usually small and mononuclear, with scanty granules or sparse granules. The bone marrow will show dyserythropiesis, small megakaryocytes, promyelocytes with sparse granules, promonocytes, hypogranular precursors, ringed sideroblasts and multinucleated normoblasts with vacuolation. Chemotherapy can be effective, but a bone marrow transplant is more effective.

4. Answer: C

Haem iron is taken to the cytoplasm where the porphyrin ring is cleaved and the iron released. Non-haem iron exists almost exclusively as insoluble ferric salts; to be absorbed, these must be reduced to the ferrous form and bound to the intestinal iron transport protein, mucosal apotransferritin. Absorption of non-haem iron is also reduced with increased intake of phytates and phosphates, so vegans are at risk of iron deficiency anaemia even if they are taking adequate iron.

Apotransferrin is a mucosal cell transporter for iron and is secreted by the liver.

5. Answer: D

Iron deficiency anaemia

Plasma transferrin receptors, plasma iron and total iron binding capacity are also reduced. Free erythrocyte zinc protoporphyrin will give an estimation of the iron level over a longer time. It helps to find the cause and how long it is been ongoing. Serum iron and ferritin levels give a clear idea of the level of iron in the system.

6. Answer: B

Iron deficiency anaemia

The oral supplementation for iron deficiency is 3 mg/kg/day, up to a maximum of 180 mg daily, which can be given as a single dose or twice per day. 9 mg of ferrous fumarate will provide 3 mg of iron. Other possible supplements include 21 mg of sodium iron edetate or 9 mg of dried ferrous sulfate. Ferrous sulfate is most commonly used. Once or twice weekly might be more effective than daily, as treatment for one day will saturate or block the intestinal absorption processes so that the next day's dose will be less well absorbed. A total of 3 months' supplement should be adopted, and close follow-up is needed with the aim of increasing the Hb level to 10 g/dl before stopping the oral treatment.

7. Answer: E

Megaloblastic anaemia

There are many causes, including inherited and acquired causes. The inherited forms are thiamine-responsive megaloblastic anaemia, folate malabsorption, methylmalonic aciduria, intrinsic factor deficiency, transcobalamin deficiency and methylenetetrahydrofolate deficiency. Acquired causes include total or subtotal gastrostomy, a vegan diet, stagnant loop syndrome, chronic tropical sprue, coeliac disease, Crohn's disease, low potassium and drugs (colchicine, phenformin, metformin and cholestyramine).

8. Answer: C

Erythropoiesis

Red cell production is at its lowest level in the 2nd week of life. The lifespan of red cells in the first 12 weeks of life will be reduced to 60–80 days in term babies and 35–45 days in preterm babies. Babies usually remain reticulocytopenic in the first 1–6 weeks of life, as erythroid activity in the bone marrow does not start to increase until 3–4 weeks of age.

9. Answer: C

Haemolysis

The causes of haemolytic anaemia in the first 6 months of life are as follows. Rh, ABO, maternal autoantibodies and drugs will cause immune haemolytics that will show within the first few hours to days after delivery. Other causes include bacterial or congenital infections, renal artery stenosis, coarctation of the aorta, large-vessel thrombi, hereditary elliptocytosis, G6PD deficiency, glucose isomerase deficiency and α-thalassaemia. Macro- or microangiopathic haemolytic anaemia can be caused by DIC.

10. Answer: B

Anaemia of prematurity

Other factors include reticulocytopenia, reduction in the level of erythropoietin level with reduction in erythropoietin response to anaemia or hypoxia, reduction in hepatic synthesis of erythropoietin, rapid growth rate and increase in blood volume, and reduced level of other haemopoietic growth factors.

11. Answer: D

Autoimmune haemolytic anaemia

Other drugs include quinine, phenacetin and sulfonamides. The mechanism is the formation of IgG and IgM antibodies directed against the medication or one of its metabolites, although IgM is very rarely the cause of haemolysis.

12. Answer: D

Inherited blood disorders

Neonates with leukaemia or other malignancy and those undergoing chemotherapy should also receive irradiated blood products. Recipients of familial blood or HLA-matched cellular products, or of solid organ or tissue transplants should be transfused only with irradiated blood products. This is also true for any child with a choanal–truncal heart defect until congenital T-cell immunodeficiency has been ruled out.

13. Answer: D

Fresh frozen plasma

Fresh frozen plasma can be used to correct overdosage with vitamin K antagonists. Fresh frozen plasma should not be used as a replacement fluid, for treatment of isolated congenital procoagulant or anticoagulant factor deficiency, for correction of hypergammaglobulinaemia, for correction or prevention of protein malnutrition, or for intravascular expansion or repletion. Fresh frozen plasma is used almost exclusively to treat or prevent clinically significant bleeding due to a deficiency of one or more plasma coagulation factors.

14. Answer: C

Vitamin K-dependent coagulation factors

The other vitamin K-dependent factors are protein S and factor X. These are all affected by warfarin, and in patients who are on warfarin and require surgery or are acutely ill or actively bleeding, the action of warfarin needs to be reversed. This is done either by modifying the warfarin, by giving vitamin K (IV or IM), by giving a plasma transfusion or, in rare situations, by giving a virus-inactivated plasma-derived prothrombin complex concentrate. Prior to surgery, warfarin should stopped for 72 hours. In severe liver diseases, there are deficiencies in the biosynthesis of antithrombin III, proteins C and S, plasminogen, antiplasmins and coagulation factors. There is also thrombocytopenia and platelet dysfunction. There is accelerated destruction of coagulation factors.

15. Answer: C

16. Answer: B

Acute lymphoblastic leukaemia

- L1 ALL is also characterized by the nucleoli being invisible or small and inconspicuous and more vesicular. The nuclear shape is regular, occasionally clefted or indented. The cells are small.
- L2 ALL is characterized by large cells, and the nuclear chromatin is variable and heterogenous in any given case, with an irregular nuclear shape and one or more nucleoli. The cytoplasm is variable, with variable basophilia and vacuolation.
- In L3 ALL, the cells are large and homogenous, the nuclear chromatin is fine and stippled, and the nucleus is regular and oval. The nucleoli are prominent and one or two in number, the cytoplasm is moderately abundant with pronounced basophilia, and cytoplasmic vacuolation is often prominent.

17–20. Answers:

17. **D:** There are no other features of Fanconi anaemia.
18. **C:** Pancreatic insufficiency is associated with Shwachman–Diamond syndrome.
19. **G:** Skin changes with an increased risk of cancer and bone marrow failure are the main characteristic features of dyskeratosis congenita.
20. **E:** The DNA repair study will be normal, and the presence of the thumb is another feature of TAR syndrome.

21–24. Answers:

21. **D:** About 80% of RVT occurs in the first month of life and sometimes in utero. It is bilateral in one-quarter of patients. Causes include perinatal asphyxia, shock, polycythaemia and cyanotic congenital heart disease. Older children usually present with haematuria, flank pain, oedema and enlarged kidneys. RVT is usually secondary to nephritic syndrome, burns, dehydration and SLE, and can be treated with heparin with supportive measures for renal failure.

22. **H:** Factor VIII activity level is reduced with haemophilia type A, while in haemophilia B factor XI is reduced. The presentation in the neonatal period is usually as a haematoma after IM injections, as a leaking umbilical cord or after circumcision. Type B usually presents later. The current treatment for type A is recombinant factor VIII. Treatment of type B is with highly purified plasma-derived product, as recombinant factor XI has not yet been licensed.

23. **C:** Lymphoblastic NHL comprises 20% of cases of NHL. It usually presents with mediastinal and nodal masses. It is usually heterogenous. It can also involve the bone, skin, thyroid and testis. The cure rate for T-cell NHL is 60–65% while that for B-cell NHL is 80–85%. Staging and management are not very different from those for other types of NHL.

24. **F:** The favourable prognostic features for ALL are age greater than 1 year and less than 6 years, WCC $<20 \times 10^9$/l, M1 marrow, chromosomal index >50, DNA index >1.16, the chromosomal translocation t(12;21) (*TEL–AML1* gene fusion) (for which the 5-year event-free survival rate is about 80%), and a response to the initial 7 days of prednisolone monotherapy, plus intrathecal methotrexate on day 1, with peripheral blasts $<1\%$. ALL can affect every organ in the body, and presentation can be different in each case. The favourable prognostic factors for relapsed treated ALL are late relapse (6–12 months from remission), extramedullary relapse, peripheral blasts at relapse of $<10 \times 10^9$, with immunotype of B-precursor ALL, the t(12;21) chromosomal translocation and response to relapse treatment within 6 weeks.

25–28. Answers:

25. E: Adenosine deaminase deficiency is an autosomal recessive condition, with 15% of cases resembling severe combined immune deficiency syndrome. Adenosine deaminase is an enzyme of the purine salvage pathway that catalyses the irreversible deanimation of adenosine and deoxyadenosine to inosine and deoxyinosine. These metabolites can then be converted into purines that can be used or removed. Failure of enzyme activation will lead to accumulation of toxic metabolites such as deoxyadenosine, which inhibits DNA synthesis. The gene is located on chromosome 20q13.4, and there are many different mutations. Measuring the enzyme will help to reach the diagnosis.

26. B, K: Wiskott–Aldrich syndrome is an X-linked condition characterized by infection, eczema and thrombocytopenia. The initial presentation is usually that of petechial rashes that increase in severity. The eczema also increases in severity from age 6 months. A bacterial infection in the form of otitis media and pneumonia can be the presenting feature, which is recurrent. Molecular genetics studies have shown that Wiskott–Aldrich syndrome is caused by a mutation in the *WASP* gene. Viral infections with HSV and EBV are common. Prophylactic antibiotics are used, with aggressive treatment of viral infection.

27. D, H: In X-linked agammaglobulinaemia, a mutation in the Bruton tyrosine kinase gene (*Btk*) on chromosome Xq22 results in failure of B-cell development, with a reduction in antibody production. These children will contract a severe infection, such as an upper or lower respiratory infection, meningitis, septicaemia or septic arthritis. They are also at risk of viral infection with coxsackie and echoviruses, as antibodies play a role in protection against these disseminated viruses. IgG replacement will be the treatment, but a bone marrow transplantation is curative.

28. F, G: Human immunodeficiency virus (HIV) 1 and 2 can present asymptomatically or with lymphadenopathy, splenomegaly, hepatomegaly, skin rashes, otitis media, repeated chest infections and failure to thrive. Parotitis is also common. Treatment of HIV infection uses combinations of three types of drugs: nucleoside analogue reverse transcriptase inhibitors (e.g. zidovudine, didanosine, lamivudine, zalcitabine and stavudine), non-nucleoside reverse transcriptase inhibitors (e.g. efavirenz and nevirapine) and protease inhibitors (e.g. ritonavir, indinavir and saquinavir). There are diffrerent regimens for different age groups, and according to the viral load and immune status of patients.

Endocrinology

BOFs

1. **The following are all true regarding steroids and thyroid hormones except:**
   A Both bind to protein receptors.
   B Both are hydrophobic.
   C Both show a rapid response through surface receptors/second-messenger system.
   D The protein binding occurs in the cytoplasm or nucleus.
   E Protein-bound receptors for these hormones are intracellular in origin.

2. **In a child who looks normal with a low growth velocity and weight above the 90th centile, which of the following may be the cause of his short stature?**
   A Cushing's syndrome
   B Chromosomal abnormalities
   C Hypothyroidism
   D Hypopituitarism
   E All of the above

3. **All of the following are true about the pituitary gland except:**
   A It is derived from the primitive pharyngeal lining.
   B Cells secreting growth hormone will be seen at 5 weeks of gestation.
   C Fetal growth hormone is higher in a 2-day-old baby.
   D Congenital hypopituitarism causes hypoglycaemia and only responds to hormone replacement.
   E Suppression of LHRH is more marked in the male fetus.

4. **All of the following are true about undescended testes except:**
   A Less than 5% of term male infants have undescended testes.
   B Human chorionic gonadotrophin can be used in infants whose testes are not in the scrotum after 1 year of age.
   C Human chorionic gonadotrophin and surgical orchidopexy cannot be used together for undescended testes.
   D Anorchia will cause high serum FSH and LH.
   E A persistent müllerian duct may be involved in gonadal dysgenesis.

5. The following are all causes of diabetes insipidus in children except:

   A Rifampicin
   B Holoprosencephaly
   C Hypokalaemia
   D Cavernous sinus aneurysm
   E Hyperphosphataemia

6. All of the following are associated with a period of excessive growth except:

   A Thyrotoxicosis
   B Pseudohypoparathyroidism
   C Simple obesity
   D Gigantism
   E Precocious puberty

7. The syndrome of inappropriate antidiuretic hormone secretion (SIADH) is characterized by all of the following except:

   A Hyponatraemia
   B Infusion of 3% saline at rate of 0.05 ml/kg/min can be given to correct electrolyte imbalance
   C Total intake of water should be restricted to 30% less than that of insensible urinary loss
   D Urinary sodium will be low
   E Serum potassium is normal

8. The following are true about puberty except:

   A It is determined by growth hormones and sex steroids.
   B Oestrogen is important for skeletal maturation and fusion of the epiphyses.
   C There is no change in IGF-I concentration through puberty.
   D IGFBP-3 levels increase mostly during puberty.
   E Delayed puberty in boys can be expressed, but for delays in secondary sexual characteristics, even an endocrinological test will be normal.

9. Pubertal delay can be caused by all of the following except:

   A Turner's syndrome
   B XY gonadal dysgenesis
   C Multiple autoimmune polyendocrinopathy syndrome
   D Anorchia
   E Steroid-resistant nephrotic syndrome

10. **The following changes all occur during normal menstruation except:**

    A Oestradiol levels rise in the mid-follicular phase.
    B The luteal phase is characterized by follicular selection, maturation and ovulation occurence.
    C In the final days of the preceding cycle, initial follicular growth occurs.
    D Follicular recruitment occurs during the first 4 days of the cycle.
    E Oestrogen concentration increases during the follicular phase.

11. **The following are all characteristic features of polycystic ovary syndrome except:**

    A Hirsutism
    B Obesity
    C Anovulation
    D Low testosterone level
    E High LH level

12. **All of the following are true about the testes except:**

    A The transabdominal phase of testicular descent is under androgen control.
    B Inguinoscrotal descent occurs around 28–35 weeks of gestation.
    C A human chorionic gonadotrophin test can distinguish between undescended testes and anorchia.
    D Orchidopexy should be performed after 6 months of age.
    E For undescended testes, there is poor success with hormonal therapy.

EMQs

13–17. From the list below, for the following cases, match the hormone(s) that are appropriate physiological parameters associated with changes in hormone concentration:

   13. A child who sleeps 9 hours per day
   14. A 13-year-old girl who has finished her pubertal spurt
   15. A child who suffers from stress and anxiety
   16. A toddler who has just had his meal
   17. A 15-year-old who has just started her menstrual cycle

Options
A Growth hormone
B Prolactin
C LH
D FSH
E Insulin
F Oestradiol
G Testosterone
H Progesterone
I   Glucagon
J IGF-I
K Adrenal steroids
L Gonadal steroids
M Cortisol

18–21. The following clinical scenarios are linked to causes of diabetes insipidus. Choose the most likely diagnosis from the list below:

   18. A 10-month-old baby presents with failure to thrive, polydipsia and polyuria. His urine osmolarity rises to 400 mosmol/l after water restriction for 6 hours. A cranial MRI shows thickening of the pituitary stalk.

   19. A 3-month-old baby is not gaining weight, and his urine osmolarity shows <100 mosmol/kg. Oxytocin is normal, but the vasopressin level is low. A genetic study shows an abnormal gene on Xq28.

   20. A 3-year-old boy is seen with a history of polydipsia and polyuria. His cranial MRI is normal, and his urine osmolarity rises to 300 mosmol/l after he is given DDAVP, as well as with a water deprivation test.

   21. A 10-year-old boy presents with dehydration. His serum sodium is 160 mmol/l and osmolarity 310 mosmol/l. His urine osmolarity is less than 100 mosmol/l. His basal plasma vasopressin is elevated at >2 pg/ml.

Options

A Nephrogenic diabetes insipidus
B X-linked familial DI
C Psychogenic diabetes insipidus
D Central diabetes insipidus
E Primary polydipsia
F Acquired polydipsia

22–25. Choose for the following scenarios the most appropriate diagnosis from the list below:

22. A 6-year-old girl presents with development of pubic hair over the last 3 months. Her height is on the 75% centile, a pelvic ultrasound is reported as normal, and LH and FSH are at prepubertal levels. The random cortisol level is 200 mmol/l, which falls within the normal range.

23. A 4-year-old girl is seen with a vaginal bleed. There are hyperpigmented patches on her neck and back, which have serrated edges. Pelvic ultrasound shows a large ovarian cyst. There is breast enlargement and a few pubic hairs.

24. A 3-year-old girl presents with lethargy, and is overweight and with developmental delay. The TSH is 12.3 mmol/l. She has also developed a vaginal bleed in the last 3 weeks. Pelvic ultrasound shows an ovarian cyst.

25. A 6-year-old boy presents with pubic hair, normal testicles, and size and height both over the 75th centile. Urinary 17-hydroxyprogesterone is high.

Options

A Adrenal tumour
B Congenital adrenal hyperplasia
C Premature adrenarche
D Hypothyroidism
E Autoimmune ovarian cyst
F McCune–Albright syndrome
G Septo-optic dysplasia
H Hydrocephalus
I Hypothalamic haematoma
J Pituitary adenoma
K Tumour secreting sex steroids
L Exogenous sources of sex steroids

26–29. Choose from the list below the most likely investigation for the following scenarios:

26. A 2-day-old baby presents with hypotonia and respiratory distress and is not feeding. His corrected calcium is reported as 3.2 mmol/l.

27. A 28-day-old girl is found to have a TSH of 20 mU/l and a T_4 of 9 μg/dl. A radionuclide scan with ^{123}I shows no uptake by thyroid tissue anywhere.

28. A 10-year-old girl presents with thyroid gland enlargement, tremors, lack of sleep, proximal muscle weakness, weight loss, inability to tolerate heat, headache and a rapid heart-beat. Her height is on the 90th centile. Her hair is fine, and there is diffused enlargement of the thyroid gland. Her T_4 is 40 μg/l, and her TSH is < 1 mU/l. TSH receptors ABC are negative.

29. A 14-year-old boy presents with enlargement of the thyroid gland. His TSH is low at 2 mU/l, his T_4 is 29 μg/l and he is positive for TSH receptors ABC. A thyroid scan indicates cold nodules and neck ultrasound indicates a solid thyroid gland.

Options

A Fine-needle aspiration of thyroid gland
B Ultrasound of the neck
C Radioisotope scan with ^{123}I
D Radioisotope scan with ^{99m}Tc pertechnetate
E Serum antibodies to Tg
F Serum microsomal antibodies to TPO
G Free T_3 level
H Urinary iodine
I TRH
J TBG
K Brain MRI
L Parathyroid hormone

Answers for Endocrinology

1. Answer: C

Intracellular receptors for hormones

Both steroids and thyroid hormones are bound to intracellular protein receptors. Both are hydrophobic, diffuse easily across the plasma membrane of their target cells and gain access to intracellular receptors that can be found in the cytoplasm or nucleus.

2. Answer: B

Short stature

Failure of physical growth could be a mark of an endocrine, systemic or genetic problem. Before performing any investigations, a detailed history and thorough clinical examination are very important. Precision anthropometry is very important for diagnosing children with short stature. A child who is short, shows slow velocity and looks thin will be suffering from a systemic chronic disease. A child who is short with dysmorphic features could have chromosomal abnormalities, not hormonal ones. A child with disproportionate short stature may have short limbs or a short back and limbs, and he/she does not need hormonal testing in most cases. Clinical examination may show achondroplasia, hypochondroplasia, metaphyseal chondroplasia or multiple epiphyseal dysplasia.

3. Answer: B

Pituitary gland

Cell secreting growth hormone will be seen at 10 weeks; at 5 weeks, cells secreting prolactin will be seen. The fetal growth hormone ACTH is higher than in a 2-day-old baby. The combination of growth hormone and cortisol deficiencies in congenital hypopituitarism will cause severe hypoglycaemia, which only responds to replacement of these two hormones. LHRH will be more suppressed in a male fetus because of testosterone.

4. Answer: C

Undescended testes

This is more likely in premature babies but less than 5% of term babies are affected, and by 1 year of age this figure should be 0.08%. Human chorionic gonadotrophin and surgical orchidopexy can be used separately or together. Incomplete descended testes may indicate the presence of an underlying gonadotrophin deficiency. Serum FSH and LH will be high in children without testes. Pelvic ultrasound and/or MRI are good investigational tools, as they may show a remnant of the müllerian duct, which is responsible for gonadal dysgenesis or persistent müllerian duct syndrome.

5. Answer: E

6. Answer: B

7. Answer: D

Syndrome of inappropriate antidiuretic hormone secretion (SIADH)

Patients with SIADH do not exhibit oedema or postural hypotension. Plasma urea, creatinine, urate and renin tend to be low and urinary sodium high. Serum aldosterone is low and serum potassium is normal. Thyroid function and morning cortisol are normal, which will exclude SIADH secondary to hypothyroidism and secondary hypoadrenalism. An infusion of 3% saline can be given to raise serum sodium by not more than 12 mmol/day up to 133–135 mmol/l, but should be used with caution. Treatment is via fluid restriction and of the underlying cause of SIADH.

8. Answer: C

9. Answer: E

Causes of pubertal delay

In boys, this can be due to undescended testes, or can follow untreated torsion of the testes or infection or trauma to the testes. In girls, it can be due to autoimmune ovarian failure or galactosaemia. In both sexes, it can be caused by chemotherapy and radiotherapy, pituitary and hypothalamic damage due to infection, tumour or trauma, Kallmann's syndrome (which is also associated with anosmia), and defects in GnRH-secreting neurones with adrenal failure and X-linked ichthyosis. Chronic diseases can also cause delay in puberty and growth arrest. Investigations in these cases can be directed at the suspected cause, but general rules should be applied in investigations, starting with baseline testing, including random steroids, LH, FSH, TFT and bone age, with pelvic ultrasound in girls.

10. Answer: B

Normal cycles in girls

The follicular phase is characterized by selection of follicles, as well as maturation and ovulation. The oestrogen concentration increases during this phase. In the mid-follicular phase, the FSH level falls, and maturation of other follicles is suppressed, with the oestradiol level rising. In the luteal phase, the level of progesterone is high, and endometrial differentiation occurs.

11. Answer: D

Polycystic ovary syndrome (PCOS)

This is characterized by disorders of menstrual function, hirsutism, obesity, hyperandrogenism and anovulation. The serum levels of testosterone and LH are high. Raised LH is not universal. The cytochrome P450 cholesterol side-chain cleavage gene (*CYP11a*), the insulin gene (*VNTR*) and the follistatin gene may all play a role in the aetiology of PCOS. Presentation is usually with hirsutism and oligomenorrhoea or menorrhoea. It usually presents early in adolescence. There is a known association of obesity, hyperinsulinaemia, insulin resistance and PCOS, and it is characterized by increased upper body mass, raised triglycerides, subnormal high-density lipoprotein (HDL) and relative glucose intolerance.

Treatment involves weight reduction and the use of progesterone therapy, or, in older adolescents, the combined oral contraceptive, which contains oestrogen and progesterone. Hirsutism can be treated by depilatory creams, waxing or electrolysis. Antandrogens are very useful for treating hirsutism.

12. Answer: A

Testes

The embryology of the testes is divided into two phases. The first is the transabdominal phase, which occurs between 10 and 15 weeks of gestation and is under the control of the anti-müllerian hormone. The testes move from the urogenital ridge to the inguinal region. The migratory inguinoscrotal phase occurs between 28 and 35 weeks of gestation and is controlled by androgens. The testes can be undescended, ectopic or retractile. A complete examination is a good investigative tool to differentiate between these. A variety of imaging techniques have been used for undescended testes, including ultrasound, CT, MRI, arteriorography and venography. It is now agreed that all of these techniques are of limited value and are less accurate than an experienced examiner. The absence of testosterone response with hCG tests is an indication of anorchia. Using hCG and GnRH in the treatment of undescended testes has been widely used, but less than one-fifth of these patients will benefit, although this approach can be used successfully for retractile testes. The risk of malignancy is high if an orchidopexy is not done within the first 2 years of life.

13–17. Answers:

   13. A, B
   14. C, D, K, L
   15. A, B, M
   16. E, I
   17. D, E, F, H

Hormonal assays

The measurement of hormones and the interpretation of results obtained can be complicated by many physiological variables. Some hormones can exhibit a very high circadian rhythm that may develop during puberty. Both protein and steroid hormones may increase during stress and exercise, and in some cases this may be difficult to interpret. Most hormones are measured in the blood using immunoassay techniques. Urine measurements can also be used, particularly for enzyme disorders, steroid biosynthesis and detecting synthetic steroids. Measuring growth hormones in urine has proven value in cases with suspected growth hormone deficiency.

18–21. Answers:

   18. D
   19. B
   20. F
   21. A

Diabetes insipidus (DI)

There are many central (pituitary) causes of DI, including genetics and congenital malformations such as midline craniofacial defects, holoprosencephaly and agenesis of the pituitary gland. Acquired causes include trauma, neoplasms (e.g. craniopharyngioma, meningioma, lymphoma, leukaemia and granuloma), infections (e.g. meningitis and encephalitis) and vascular causes (e.g. cavernous sinus aneurysm). Hypoxic encephalopathy can also cause DI. In many cases, no cause can be found. Nephrogenic DI can be genetic (X-linked or autosomal recessive). Acquired DI can be caused by drugs (including lithium, demeclocycline and cisplatin), hypercalciuria, sickle cell disease and trait, and granulomas, and can also be idiopathic. Primary polydipsia can be acquired, as in iatrogenic and psychogenic forms; abnormal thirst may be due to granulomas, infection, head trauma, lithium or multiple sclerosis.

   In cases of suspected DI, the diagnosis can be verified by measuring urine volume, osmolarity and creatinine content of a 24-hour urine collection. If these are normal, there is no need for further testing. If they are abnormal, a water deprivation test should be done. If fluid restriction does not result in concentration of the urine at >300 mosmol/kg, with Na reaching 146 mmol/l, then primary polydipsia and partial vasopressin deficiency can be ruled out. The distinction between central and nephrogenic DI can be made by injecting 1–2 u of aqueous vasopressin (Pitressin) or 1–2 μg of desmopressin (DDAVP) and repeating the measurements of urine osmolarity 1–2 hours later. A rise in urine osmolarity by 50% is diagnostic of central DI, while a rise of <50% will indicate nephrogenic DI. Treatment of central DI is with desmopressin, which can be given IV, intranasally or orally. Treatment of nephrogenic DI is according to the cause. Primary polydipsia can be treated with education and behavioural management. Desmopressin is contraindicated in these cases.

22–25. Answers:

22. C
23. F
24. D
25. B

Assessment of children with precocious puberty

Assessment of a child with possible precocious puberty should first include history, weight and height. Tanner pubertal staging should be performed accurately in both boys and girls. If there is an increase in height velocity then bone age will be of value in assessing these children. In the case of gonadal steroid oversecretion, girls will have breast enlargement and boys will have testicular enlargement. In these cases, all girls should have cerebral imaging, preferably an MRI scan. In girls without neurological signs, the chance of finding a lesion is very low. In girls, a pelvic ultrasound will help considerably. In puberty, there is an increase in ovarian volume and in follicle size and number, and the shape of the uterus changes from tubular to pear-shaped. The same changes are seen in central precocious puberty, but not in premature thelarche.

In central precocious puberty, the sex steroids LH and FSH will be low in random testing. The response to GnRH stimulation is the same as in normal puberty, with LH predominant. In gonadotrophin-independent puberty, the response to GnRH is flat, as the feedback suppression is elevated by sex steroid concentration. In cases of McCune–Albright syndrome, a radioisotope bone scan will detect the olyostotic fibrous dysplasia. Serum adrenal androgen levels are not helpful in confirming a diagnosis of premature adrenarche.

26–29. Answers:

26. L
27. B
28. B
29. A

Nephrology

BOFs

1. In acute renal failure, the urine-to-plasma creatinine ratio is:

   A <5
   B <10
   C <15
   D >40
   E <20

2. The following all cause sustained hypertension in children except:

   A Renal artery stenosis
   B Conn's disease
   C Nephrotic syndrome
   D Essential hypertension
   E Polycystic kidneys

3. The following drugs can cause haematuria except:

   A Sulfonamides
   B Aspirin
   C Ceftriaxone
   D Indometacin (indomethacin)
   E Amitriptyline

4. A 4 month old baby girl was born at 28/40. Urea is 40 mmol/l, creatinine 350 mmol/l and urine output 1 ml/kg/h. Her sodium is 127 mmol/l and potassium 5.7 mmol/l. Her clotting is normal, and conjugated bilirubin is 30 mmol/l, with normal ALT. The urine osmolarity is <400 mosmol/l, and urinary sodium 75 mmol/l. The child is very oedematous, with a mean arterial blood pressure of 26 mmHg. What is the most likely cause of her oedema?

   A Congenital nephrotic syndrome
   B Acute renal failure
   C Chronic renal failure
   D Hypothyroidism
   E Hepatic failure

5. In metabolic acidosis, decreased acid excretion can be caused by all of the following except:

   A Early salicylate poisoning
   B Distal renal tubular acidosis
   C Acute renal failure
   D Chronic renal failure
   E Carbonic anhydrase inhibitors

6. The most common causes of polyuria and polydipsia in children include the following except:

   A Chronic renal failure
   B Diabetes mellitus
   C Psychogenic
   D Behavioural
   E Urinary tract infection

7. A 10-year-old girl presents with soreness of her vulval area, itching and dysuria. There is no growth on urine culture, nor is there any vaginal discharge. Her stool is negative for infection and blood. Her parents say that there is a strong unpleasant smell from the child's underpants. What is the most likely diagnosis?

   A Urinary tract infection
   B Child sexual abuse
   C Vulvovaginitis
   D Eczema
   E None of the above

8. In IgA nephropathy, all of the following are true except:

   A The serum C3 level is normal.
   B The immune complex is positive on electron microscopy.
   C The serum C4 level is high.
   D Haematuria is common.
   E IgA serum level may be elevated.

9. A 7-year-old boy is admitted with acute diarrhoea and vomiting over the last 48 hours. He is 10% dehydrated, and his urine output is less than 0.5 ml/kg/h over the last 24 hours. His potassium is 7 mmol/l, urea 45 mmol/l and creatinine 300 mmol/l. His acute renal failure is worsening and his potassium is rising. Which of the following should be excluded in the management of his hyperkalaemia before commencing dialysis?

   A IV infusion of glucose and insulin
   B IV infusion of 7.5% bicarbonate
   C IV corticosteroids
   D IV infusion of salbutamol
   E Rectal ion exchange resins

10. Anaemia associated with chronic renal failure is caused by:

A Reduced red cell production
B Increase in production of testosterone
C Iron depletion
D Iron toxicity from excessive transfusion
E Splenomegaly

11. A 3-year-old child presents with microscopic haematuria and dysuria. Renal ultrasound shows one calculi in his bladder. He has passed three stones in his urine in the past. His brother suffered from recurrent renal stones, but responded very well to treatment with D-penicillamine. What is the most likely diagnosis?

A Cystinosis
B Cystinuria
C Primary hyperparathyroidism
D Idiopathic hypocalcaemia
E Xanthinuria

12. The following are all true about infantile polycystic renal disease in older children except:

A There is progressive renal failure.
B It is an autosomal recessive disorder.
C It is associated with severe hypertension.
D Portal hypertension is a well-recognized feature.
E There are respiratory problems.

13. Infants with horseshoe kidneys are likely to have:

A Hypertension
B Renal colic
C Features of Turner's syndrome
D Renal calculi
E Renal artery stenosis

14. In newborn babies, acute urinary obstruction is due to all of the following except:

A Posterior urethral valve
B Spinal cord compression
C Pelvic teratoma
D Rhabdomyosarcoma
E Urethrocele

EMQs

15–18. From the following scenarios, choose the most appropriate diagnosis from the list below:

15. A 3-year-old girl presents with abdominal pain, dysuria, bed-wetting, haematuria and a urinary tract infection. MCUG shows no reflux. DTPA shows delay in excretion of isotopes from the left kidney, with an increase in flow in response to furosemide (frusemide).

16. A 3-year-old boy has had increased swelling of his legs, abdomen and face over the last 10 days. The urine shows proteinuria and haematuria, and the blood pressure is 110/70 mmHg. He has gained 3 kg in the last 10 days.

17. A 10-year-old child presents with macroscopic haematuria for the second time in the last 3 months. Urine culture is negative and renal ultrasound is normal. C3 and C4 levels and urine microscopy for casts and protein are negative. His renal biopsy shows mesangial deposition of IgA and a normal basement membrane.

18. A 3-week-old male infant has a history of diarrhoea for 3 days. His urine shows gross haematuria, with one plus protein and urine output less than 1 ml/kg/h. He is diagnosed as having acute renal failure from a biochemical test, and management of renal failure is started. His left kidney is palpable with a normal appearance.

Options
A Renal vein thrombosis
B Nephrotic syndrome
C Acute glomerulonephritis
D Urticaria
E Renal failure
F PUJ obstruction
G Polycystic kidney disease
H Posterior urethral valve
I Renal agenesis
J Hydronephrosis
K Alport's syndrome
L Post-Henoch–Schönlein nephritis
M Berger's disease
N Basement membrane nephropathy
O Glomerulonephritis
P Renal tumour
Q Left renal vein thrombosis
R Hydronephrosis of the left kidney
S Infantile polycystic kidney disease
T Congenital nephrotic syndrome

19–21. For the following scenarios, choose the most appropriate management plan for each case from the list below:

19. A 6-year-old boy is referred with a history of bed-wetting. His urine shows no growth, and he is doing well at school. The GP organized an ultrasound scan of his kidneys, which was reported as normal. He lives with his mother and 10-year-old brother. His father is in prison and his mother has a new partner.

20. A 4-year-old child presents with a diagnosis of passing calculi in his urine on many occasions. He is developmentally delayed, with thick upper lips, a depressed nasal bridge and prominent maxilla. He is very sociable and is very popular in the nursery. His ultrasound shows multiple small renal calculi, and his father says that he has problems with his heart on the right side (William's Syndrome).

21. A 2-year-old boy presents with lethargy and fever and is sleepy. His urine output is less than 0.5 ml/kg/h and his serum potassium 6.9 mmol/l.

Options
A   Refer to an enuresis clinic
B   Start on treatment (desmopressin nasal spray)
C   Repeat renal ultrasound and urine analysis
D   Refer to a psychologist
E   Start star achievement cards
F   Low calcium intake
G   Intravenous insulin
H   Oral calcium gluconate
I   Intravenous calcitonin
J   Intravenous salbutamol

Answers for Nephrology

1. Answer: E

The urine-to-plasma creatinine ratio is >40 in prerenal failure. In acute renal failure, the urine sodium is >40 mmol/l, the fractional excretion of filtered sodium is >1, urine osmolarity is <350 mosmol/l and the urine-to-plasma urea nitrogen ratio is <3.

2. Answer: C

Hypertension

In children, this can be caused by renal nephropathies, renal vascular disease, aortic coarctation, glomerulonephritis, corticosteroid excess (e.g. Conn's disease, Cushing's syndrome and congenital adrenal hyperplasia), low renin, haemolytic uraemic syndrome, phaeochromocytoma, neuroblastoma and nephroblastoma. There are also idiopathic cases.

3. Answer: C

Haematuria

Haematuria can be caused by glomular problems such as thin basement membrane diseases, Alport's syndrome, IgA nephropathy, haemolytic uraemic syndrome, post-infectious glomerulonephritis, membranoproliferative glomerulonephritis, lupus nephritis and anaphylactoid purpura (Henoch–Schönlein purpura). Other non-glomerular causes include fever, strenuous exercise, drugs/toxins, foreign bodies, mechanical trauma, urinary tract infection, hypercalciuria/urolithiasis, sickle cell disease/trait, coagulopathy, tumours, anatomical abnormalities (hydronephrosis, polycystic kidney disease and vascular malformations), masturbation and menstruation.

4. Answer: C

Chronic renal failure (CRF)

CRF in children can be progressive and be caused by systemic hypertension, acute insults from nephrotoxins or decreased perfusion, proteinuria, increased renal ammoniagenesis with interstitial injury, hyperlipidaemia, hyperphosphataemia with calcium phosphate deposition, and decreased levels of nitrous oxide. The manifestation of CRF is hyperkalaemia, which usually develops when the glomerular filtration rate GFR falls to less than 20–25 cm^3/min because of the decreased ability of the kidneys to excrete potassium. It can be observed sooner in patients who ingest a potassium-rich diet or if serum aldosterone levels are low. Metabolic acidosis is often mixed, with the anion gap generally not higher than 20 mEq/l. In CRF, the kidneys are unable to produce enough ammonia in the proximal tubules to excrete the endogenous acid into the urine in the form of ammonium ion. In very advanced CRF, accumulation of phosphates, sulfates and other organic anions causes the small anion gap. Extracellular volume expansion and total-body volume overload result from failure of sodium and free-water excretion. These usually intensify when the GFR falls to <10–15 cm^3/min and when all compensatory mechanisms have become exhausted. Patients usually present with peripheral, rather than pulmonary, oedema. This can happen even with a higher GFR, as an excess of sodium and water intake can result in a similar picture if the ingested amounts of sodium and water exceed the potential excretion of the usual amount. Normochromic normocytic anaemia principally develops from decreased renal synthesis of erythropoietin, which is responsible for stimulation of bone marrow for red cell production. As the GFR decreases, the condition becomes more difficult to treat, and no reticulocyte response occurs. RBC lifespan is reduced, and the tendency to bleed increases as a result of uraemia-induced platelet dysfunction. Secondary hyperparathyroidism develops because of hypocalcaemia and hyperphosphataemia. The latter is a result of the inability of the kidneys to excrete the excess dietary intake, while the hypocalcaemia is caused primarily by decreased intestinal calcium absorption because of low plasma calcitriol levels and possibly as a result of calcium binding to elevated serum levels of phosphate. Renal osteodystrophy will develop because of all these changes. These lesions develop in patients with severe CRF and are common in those with end-stage renal disease (ESRD). Osteomalacia and dynamic bone disease are the two other lesions observed. Dialysis-related amyloidosis from β_2-microglobulin accumulation in patients who have required chronic dialysis for at least 8–10 years is another form of bone disease that manifests with cysts at the ends of long bones. Other manifestations of uraemia in ESRD are pericarditis, encephalopathy that can progress to coma and death, peripheral neuropathy, restless leg syndrome, GI symptoms such as anorexia, nausea, vomiting and diarrhoea, skin manifestations such as dry skin, pruritus and ecchymosis, fatigue, increased somnolence, failure to thrive, malnutrition, erectile dysfunction, decreased libido, amenorrhea, and platelet dysfunction with a tendency to bleeding.

5. Answer: A

Salicylate poisoning

Salicylates stimulate the respiratory centre, leading to hyperventilation and respiratory alkalosis. However, respiratory alkalosis may be transient in children, so that metabolic acidosis may occur early in the course. Salicylates also interfere with the Krebs cycle, limit production of ATP and increase lactate production, leading to ketosis and a wide-anion-gap metabolic acidosis. Patients with mixed acid–base disturbances have been found to have normal-anion-gap metabolic acidosis; therefore, normal-anion-gap acidosis does not exclude salicylates.

6. Answer: A

Polyuria and polydipsia

Polyuria and polydipsia are associated with diabetes insipidus (DI). There are idiopathic and familial forms of DI (both of which are very rare). It can be inherited as an autosomal dominant disorder, and mutations involving AVP/neurophysin gene have been identified as occurring after neurosurgery or trauma. Primary intracranial tumours causing DI include craniopharyngioma and pineal tumours. Possible causes also include other malignancies (e.g. lung cancer, lymphoma and leukaemia), hypoxic encephalopathy, infiltrative disorders (histocytosis X and sarcoidosis), anorexia nervosa, and vascular lesions such as arteriovenous malformations or aneurysms.

7. Answer: C

Vulvovaginitis

Vulvovaginitis will produce local pain, burning or itching, and external dysuria with a strong unpleasant smell from the genital area or from the child's underpants. A UTI can produce a similar strong smell. During the examination, the child must be relaxed and an explanation should be given for the examination. NAI, foreign bodies and threadworms should be ruled out. Poor hygiene is the most common cause, along with chemicals, nylon, eczema, scabies, fungal infections and trauma. Swabs must be taken. Avoidance of any irritants, good hygiene and any barrier creams will help. There is no need for steroids.

8. Answer: C

IgA nephropathy

The pathogenesis of IgA nephropathy remains unclear. The characteristic pathological findings are immunofluorescence microscopy of granular deposits of IgA and complement 3 (C3) in the glomular mesangium. These findings suggest that this disease occurs because of the deposition of circulating immune complexes, leading to activation of the complement cascade. In some cases there is an association of IgA nephropathy with syndromes that affect the respiratory or gastrointestinal tracts, such as coeliac disease, suggesting that IgA nephropathy is a disease of the mucosal immune system. Haematuria worsens during or after upper respiratory tract or gastrointestinal tract infections, which support its origin being mucosal.

IgA antibodies cannot activate complement through the classic pathway; studies have shown that the alternative pathway can activate complement. Serum IgA levels are elevated in approximately 50% of patients with IgA nephropathy, but that increase is unlikely to play a role in the pathogenesis of the disease because markedly elevated IgA levels are observed in patients with AIDS who do not have IgA nephropathy. However, IgA is probably accumulated and deposited because of a systemic abnormality rather than a defect intrinsic to the kidney.

9. Answer: C

Management of hyperkalaemia

10% calcium gluconate and dialysis can be used to lower potassium in acute renal failure.

10. Answer: A

Anaemia in chronic renal failure (CRF)

Anaemia in CRF is due to decreased red cell survival time and reduced red cell production as a result of a deficiency in renal erythropoietin. Splenic sequestration for RBCs can also cause anaemia. There is no role for iron supplements for patients with anaemia secondary to CRF unless iron deficiency anaemia has been proved by laboratory testing. Regular transfusions, splenectomy and exogenous testosterone for postpubertal patients can be used to treat anaemia, with other measures to treat chronic renal failure, including renal transplantation.

11. Answer: B

Cystinuria

Cystinuria is characterized by excessive secretion of the dibasic amino acids cystine, ornithine, arginine and lysine, with the same transport effect being found in the gastrointestinal tract. It is inherited as an autosomal recessive disorder. Stones can be prevented by maintaining a high urine flow and alkalizing the urine. If all fails and the patient still forms stones, D-penicillamine is effective in preventing further stones.

12. Answer: E

Infantile polycystic renal disease in older children

Renal failure usually develops in the 2nd year of life, with renal enlargement and vomiting. Blood pressure will be high and may lead to congestive heart failure. Portal hypertension will not present before the age of 5 years.

13. Answer: C

Horseshoe kidneys

Horseshoe kidneys are more common in males, and are associated with Turner's syndrome. The condition is usually asymptomatic. It can sometimes present as an infection, reflux or obstructive uropathy. Those affected are prone to hydronephrosis.

14. Answer: D

Acute urinary obstruction

The causes of acute urinary obstruction in the newborn period also include traumatic delivery and prolapsing urethrocele in females; it may also be temporary, with no obvious cause. In older children, it can be due to a posterior urethral valve in males, trauma in both males and females, rhabdomyosarcoma in males, prolapsing urethrocele is both males and females, and meatal polyps in males.

15–18. Answers:

15. F: PUJ obstruction is the most common cause of hydronephrosis; it is more common in males. In newborn babies, it can present as an abdominal mass, with vomiting and failure to thrive. Haematuria and hypertension may be associated symptoms. Abdominal ultrasound and intravenous pyelography are the investigations to confirm the diagnosis. Surgical intervention can be performed early to preserve kidney function.

16. C: The presentation of acute glomerulonephritis can be typical with facial swelling followed by lower limb swelling and passage of dark red urine. Hypertension may be noted, and is present in the majority of hospitalized children. Some may present with tachypnoea and dyspnoea due to pulmonary congestion or the presence of pleural effusion. Urine will show numerous red and white cells and less proteinuria. There will be red cell casts, which are considered as glomerular leaking in these cases. The C3 level will be low, and C4 can be low (but not in the majority of cases). Bed rest, furosemide (frusemide) and control of hypertension are used as management tools, after consultation with nephrologists.

17. M: Berger's disease (mesangial IgA nephritis) is more common in boys and can be familial. It commonly presents as haematuria followed by an upper respiratory tract infection. Abdominal pain is common, while other patients just have red urine. Haematuria can start as microscopic then become macroscopic. Only a small group progress to renal nephritis. The renal biopsy finding on immunofluorescence is of granular deposits of IgA in the mesangium of the glomerulus, which is associated with IgG and C3.

18. Q: More than three-quarters of cases of left renal vein thrombosis occur in the first month of life, with normal kidneys at birth. It is associated with gross haematuria, oliguria, renal failure and a history of diarrhoea. Proteinuria is rare, and thrombocytopenia may present. The infants of diabetic mothers with hypernatraemic dehydration and hypoxic ischaemic encephalopathy will be at high risk of getting renal vein thrombosis. Children can be managed conservatively, and a nephrectomy is not indicated.

19–21. Answers:

19. **E:** The management of enuresis starts with star achievement cards. If these do not work, use oral or nasal desmopressin. An alarm can also be used before turning on medication. Specialist enuresis clinics supported by specialist nurses, paediatricians and psychologists are sometimes also needed.

20. **F:** Hypercalcaemia can be managed by low calcium and vitamin D intake – but watch out for rickets. Intravenous calcitonin can be used in patients with hypocalcaemia secondary to malignancy.

21. **G, J:** Hyperkalaemia can be managed with 10% calcium gluconate IV; 7.5% sodium bicarbonate IV can also be used. Salbutamol infusions are used most frequently. IV insulin with glucose should be used if the others fail. Dialysis will be the last resort if the child's health deteriorates.

Rheumatology; Bone and Joint Diseases

BOFs

1. The following are causes of limping in a four-year-old child except:

   A Perthes' disease
   B Slipped femoral epiphysis
   C Juvenile chronic arthritis
   D Discitis
   E Osteomyelitis

2. The following are true about talipes equinovarus except:

   A It can be associated with myelodysplasia.
   B The congenital form is usually not associated with any other deformities.
   C It can be bilateral in 50% of cases of the congenital form.
   D It occurs in 40–50% of offspring of affected parents.
   E Serial plaster casting is one form of treatment.

3. In developmental dysplasia of the hips (DDH), the following are true except:

   A Dislocation occurs after delivery.
   B 20% of cases are familial.
   C 50–60% of breech presentation babies will have DDH.
   D A Barlow test is performed by stabilizing the pelvis and dislocating unstable hip with the other hand.
   E Babies aged 1–6 months will benefit from a Pavlik harness only.

4. All of the following are true in Perthes' disease except:

   A It affects males only.
   B It usually presents with pain in the anterior thigh, with a limp.
   C The capital femoral epiphysis will stop growing.
   D Children under 6 years of age need be observed only.
   E Periodic stretching or abduction and bed rest is another form of treatment.

5. The following are causes of back pain in children except:

   A Ankylosing spondylitis
   B Spinal epidural abscess
   C Pancreatitis
   D Appendicitis
   E Schaumann's syndrome

6. The major problems associated with different skeletal dysplasias include the following except:

   A Short stature: spondyloepiphyseal dysplasia congenita
   B Club feet: diastrophic dysplasia
   C Fractures: achondroplasia
   D Myopias and cataracts: Stickler's syndrome
   E Spinal curvature: metatrophic dysplasia

7. The most common non-lethal dwarfing condition is:

   A Chondroplasia punctata
   B Achondroplasia
   C Ellis–van Creveld syndrome
   D Osteogenesis imperfecta type I
   E Diastrophic dysplasia

8. The following are features of inherited osteoporosis except:

   A Only two forms have been identified.
   B The severe form is characterised by macrocephaly, hepato-splenomegaly, deafness and blindness.
   C Most symptoms are due to failure to remodel growing bones.
   D There is no cranial nerve involvement.
   E A generalized increase in bone density is a common feature.

9. The following are related to each subtype of osteogenesis imperfecta except:

   A Type I: blue sclera
   B Type II: multiple intrauterine fractures
   C Type III: microcephaly and triangular face
   D Type IV: bowing of legs
   E Type I: Frequent fractures

10. The following symptoms may be suggestive of rheumatic disease except:

   A Fever: systemic juvenile rheumatoid arthritis
   B Arthralgia: dermatomyositis
   C Weakness: juvenile rheumatoid arthritis
   D Chest pain: systemic lupus erythematosus
   E Back pain: spondyloarthropathy

11. The following specific antinuclear antibodies and their associations are correct except:

A Histone: drug-related lupus
B Ro/SSA: congenital heart block
C La/SSB: Sjögren's syndrome
D Ribonucleoprotein: scleroderma
E Sm: SLE

12. The following all cause foot pain in a 7-year-old child except:

A Juvenile rheumatoid arthritis
B Ewing's sarcoma
C Tarsal coalition
D Achilles tendonitis
E Hypermobile flatfoot

13. The following are common causes of back pain in children except:

A Hip–pelvic anomalies
B Discitis
C Anklosing spondylitis
D Kyphosis
E Acute lymphoblastic leukaemia

14. In torticollis, the following are the most likely causes for a child presenting to a paediatrician except:

A Visual disturbances
B Cervical cord tumour
C Gastroesophageal reflux
D Hemivertebrae
E Retropharyngeal abscess

15. The following are all lethal neonatal dwarfisms and are incompatible with life except:

A Thantophiric dysplasia
B Congenital osteoporosis
C Metatrophic dwarfism
D Achondroplasia punctuate
E Osteogenesis imperfecta type II

16. The following syndromes are associated with polydactyly except:

A Trisomy 13
B Trisomy 21
C Rubinstein–Taybi syndrome
D Carpenter's syndrome
E Ellis–van Creveld syndrome

EMQs

17–21. Choose for the following scenarios the most appropriate diagnosis from the list below:

17. A 12-year-old girl presents with a history of joint stiffening in the morning and feeling tired after school, with some joint pains in her lower limbs. On examination, her left knee is warm and swollen. The erythrocyte sedimentation rate is 55, and C-reactive protein is 70 mg/l. The white cell count is normal, with a high platelet count.

18. A 2-year-old boy presents with a fever and loss of appetite. He is miserable, complaining of pain in his neck, and has not been able to walk over the last 3 days. The joints in his legs are all swollen and hot, and he has neck stiffness. The spleen is 3 cm.

19. A 14-year-old boy presents with back pain and pain in both ankles and left knee. When he bends forward, his lower spine remains straight. There is localized tenderness around the left foot.

20. A 4-year-old girl presents with difficulty in going upstairs and leg pains. She is always tired, feels hot and has had some weight loss. The family doctor has seen her on several occasions for eczema that appears on her face and hands. It will disappear and come back within days, even without treatment. The muscle enzyme is 1500 mmol/l, and ESR is 90, with thrombocytosis. Lactate dehydrogenase is high, as is ANA.

21. A 15-year-old boy presents with painful recurrent mouth ulcers over the last 2 years. He has also presented with painful swellings on his shins (legs) on two occasions and is complaining of pains in his joints (ankles, hips, elbows and shoulders). There is lower motor neurone 7th nerve palsy that started to occur in the last 24 hours. ESR is high, and ANA and specific ANA are negative.

Options
A JCA
B Pauciarticular-onset JRA
C Polyarticular-onset JRA
D JD
E SLE
F Oligo JRA
G Systemic JRA
H Behçet's disease
I Sjögren's syndrome
J Postinfectious arthritis
K Ankylosing spondylitis
L Scleroderma
M Henoch–Schönlein purpura
N Polyarthritis nodosa

22–26. For the following conditions, choose the most appropriate treatments from the list below:

22. A 3-year-old child is diagnosed with pauciarticular-onset JCA. His ESR is 60, and an X-ray of his joints shows soft tissue swellings. Both eyes are normal.
23. A 13-year-old girl presents with weakness, chest infection and joint swelling in her lower limbs. Antinuclear antibodies are positive, and double-strand DNA is strongly positive. Her blood pressure is 140/80 mmHg.
24. A 16-year-old girl is diagnosed with scleroderma presenting as painful fingertips with colour changes over the last 3 years. She has recently started to have abdominal pain, and her blood pressure is 135/75 mmHg.
25. A 7-year-old child presents with purpuric rashes over the lower limbs, painful joints (mainly the ankles) and abdominal pain. FBC, ESR, C-reactive protein and clotting screen are all within normal ranges.
26. A 10-year-old boy presents with severe abdominal pain, fever and loss of weight over the last 2 months. The diagnosis of polyarthritis nodosa is made by biopsy of the sural nerve, which shows vasculitis. This is confirmed by coeliac angiography, which shows aneurysms in multiple vessels.

Options
A Cyclophosphamide
B Corticosteroids
C Aspirin
D NSAIDs
E Ibuprofen
F Cyclosporine
G Azathioprin
H Intravenous immunoglobulin
I Methotrexate
J Nifedepine
K Captopril
L Enalapril
M Hydroxychloroquine
N Warfarin

27–31. The following scenarios concern children presented with limping. Choose the most appropriate diagnosis from the list below:

27. A 15-month-old toddler has just started walking, but his parents have noticed that he is limping. He is afebrile and is not in pain when his hips are examined. The right leg is shorter than the left, with limitation of hip abduction. There is also waddling with lordosis and toe-walking. X-ray of his hips shows the bony roof of the right acetabulum as quite oblique, with the beginning of a false acetabulum and a displaced right femur laterally and superior.

28. A 10-year-old girl presents with limping and pain in the anterior thigh, and is walking with an antalgic gait, mild restriction of abduction of the left hip and mild restriction of internal rotation. X-ray of the left hip shows early fragmentation, a collapsed femoral head and osteopenia.

29. A 4-year-old girl presents with a waddling-like gait, and her mother has noticed that her spine is not straight. CNS examination reveals no abnormalities, and spinal X-ray AP and lateral shows scoliosis at the level of thoracic vertebrae from 4 to 10 to the left, with an angle of less than 30°. MRI of the spine shows no bony lesions.

30. A 12-year-old boy presents with back pain over the last 2 months and has visited his family doctor a few times with no improvement. He says that his thigh muscle keeps having spasms. There is limitation of lumbar flexibility, with sacral kyphosis and defects in the pars interarticularis as well as superior and inferior articular facets of a vertebral body on spinal X-ray and MRI.

31. A 27-month-old boy is brought to A&E, as he refuses to walk anymore. He was playing with his brother about 3 hours ago. There is soft swelling on his left leg just midway between the knee and ankle joints. It is tender and warm at that site. X-ray of the leg does not show any abnormalities on tibia, fibula or femur. The child is admitted, observed and discharged home with a long-leg cast, and 2 weeks later the x-ray shows subperiosteal new bone formation on the left tibia.

Options
A   Osteomyelitis
B   Septic arthritis
C   Spondylosis
D   Perthes' disease
E   Slipped capital femoral epiphysis
F   Discitis
G   Congenital scoliosis
H   Toddler fracture
I   Congenital kyphosis
J   Transient monoarticular synovitis
K   Developmental dysplasia of the hip
L   Hemiplegic cerebral palsy

Answers for Rheumatology; Bone and Joint Diseases

1. Answer: B

Limping in children

There are many other causes, including septic arthritis, trauma, neoplasms and transient synovitis of the hips. Slipped femoral epiphysis usually occurs in the teenage group only. These all cause antalgic gait.

2. Answer: D

Talipes equinovarus

There are four forms of clubfoot: congenital (which is usually an isolated abnormality), variable rigidity of the foot, mild calf atrophy, and mild hypoplasia of the tibia and fibula. It is more common in males (2:1), with a 3% recurrence rate for subsequent siblings if one is affected, and 20–30% of offspring of affected parents are themselves affected. Hind foot equinus, midfoot and hind foot varus, forefoot abduction, and variable rigidity all occur because of dislocation of the talonavicular joints. Initial treatment is conservative, and includes taping, use of malleable splints and serial plaster casts, and a significant number of children later require surgery. The other two types include teratogenic forms due to myelodysplasia or arthrogryposis multiplex congenital syndrome. The third type is positional talipes.

3. Answer: C

Dysplasia of the hips

The hips are rarely dislocated, but are rather dislocatable, so dislocation tends to occur after delivery, although the exact time is still controversial. Generalized ligamentous laxity is a related factor in most cases. About 60% of children with dislocated hips are firstborns, and 30–50% were in the breech position. The Barlow test is a provocative test to dislocate an unstable hip. It is performed by stabilizing the pelvis with one hand, flexing, adducting the apposite hip and applying posterior force. If the hip is dislocatable, it is usually felt. The management is different for each age group. Pavlik harnesses are the treatment of choice for infants between 1–6 months of age. Babies of 6–18 months are managed with surgical closed reduction as the major method of treatment. Open reduction is performed for those over 18 months. At birth or within the first month, management is by maintaining the hips in a flexion–abduction position (human position).

4. Answer: A

Perthes' disease

This is bilateral in 20% of children, and the male-to-female ratio is 4 : 1. It is a vascular necrosis of the capital femoral epiphysis (CFE). Presentation is usually with a painless limb. An X-ray should be taken anterior–posterior and laterally of the pelvis to reach the diagnosis. The X-ray will show a CFE that will stop growing, subchondral fracture, resorption (fragmentation), reossification, and healed or residual stages. Treatment can consist of just observation and regular follow-up, aiming to eliminate hip irritability, to restore hip motion and to prevent collapse of the CFE and extrusion or subluxation with the spherical femoral head. The intermittent stretching and abduction position with bed rest is another treatment if the first is not achievable. Above the age of 6 years, non-surgical abduction casts should be applied or pelvic or femoral osteotomies used.

5. Answer: D

Back pain in children

Back pain in children is unusual, and a careful history and examination should be performed. The pain can be mechanical or psychogenic. Discitis is common before the age of 6 years. Pyogenic infections (e.g. tuberculosis), should be excluded. Pyelonephritis can be the cause – but not appendicitis. Connective tissue disorders, including Reiter's disease, JCA and psoriatic arthritis, can also be causes.

Spondylolysis is common in the adolescent group. Scoliosis is another cause, with hip anomalies and herniated discs. Vertebral stress fractures and any bone tumours should be ruled out. Leukaemia is a very rare cause. Conversion reaction and juvenile osteoporosis are the least of causes.

6. Answer: C

Skeletal dysplasia

This is a group of disorders that are genetically inherited together with a clinically heterogenous group of disorders of skeletal development and growth.

Achondroplasia is not associated with frequent fractures. It is characterized by disproportionately short stature with autosomal dominant inheritance, but there are many new mutations. *FGFR3* gene mutation is commonly associated with achondroplasia. It is associated with hydrocephalus, deafness and malocclusion of the mouth. There is normal intelligence in the majority of cases. Osteogenesis imperfecta is characterized by frequent fractures, and inheritance is variable according to subtypes. Vermian bones on the skull is one of the criteria and can be seen on X-ray. Blue sclera is another association, but not with all subtypes.

7. Answer: A

Non-lethal dwarfing

Other common types include osteogenesis imperfecta types III and IV and spondyloepiphyseal dysplasia congenita; less common types include Langer's mesomelic dysplasia and metotrophic dysplasia.

8. Answer: D

Osteoporosis

The two forms are autosomal dominant and recessive. They have been genetically mapped to chromosomes 1p21 11q12–13 respectively. The severe form is also characterized by severe anaemia with diffused bone sclerosis, cranial neuropathy, failure to thrive and anaemia. This happens in infancy, and children may die during that period. The dominant form is less severe and less frequent. Patients can survive into adult life. Bone marrow transplantation is successful in some cases.

9. Answer: C

Osteogenesis imperfecta

There are only four types of osteogenesis imperfecta. Type I is the most common and is characterized by blue sclera in most cases, recurrent fractures in childhood and hearing loss. It is divided into subtypes A and B and type IV. It depends on the presence or absence of dentinogenesis. In type II, infants may be stillborn, with evidence of extreme fragility of tissues and bones or in the frog leg position with multiple bone fractures in utero and dark blue–grey sclera. Type III is the severe form. In utero fractures are common, with low birthweight and height. The sclera ranges from white to blue. Type IV demonstrates bowing of the legs and fractures in utero or after manipulation. The fracture rate decreases after puberty.

10. Answer: C

Rheumatic disease

Arthralgia is pain in the joints when trying to use them in active or passive movement. This occurs in SLE, JRA and JD, as well as in other, non-rheumatic, conditions. Weakness is mainly associated with dermatomyositis. Malar rashes are seen with SLE and photosensitive dermatitis. Chest pain from pericarditis is seen with SLE and JRA.

11. Answer: D

Antinuclear antibodies (ANAs)

An antinuclear antibody test is a screening test, with specific ANAs being found in particular diseases. Sd is specific for scleroderma and Ro/SSA for annular erythema, Sjögren's syndrome and congenital heart block. La/SSB is specific for Sjögren's syndrome, while Pm-Sd is specific for sclerodermato-myositis. Ribonucleoprotein is specific for mixed connective tissue diseases.

12. Answer: D

Foot pain in children

There are many other things that can cause pain in children, including poorly fitting shoes, Sever's disease, a foreign body, trauma and puncture wounds.

13. Answer: D

Back pain in children

Inflammatory causes are the most common that need to be ruled out; this include discitis, osteomyelitis, abscesses, pyelonephritis and pancreatitis. Reiter's disease and JRA, ankylosing spondylitis and psoriatic diseases need to be excluded, as treatment will help in reducing the pain. Neoplastic, mechanical and developmental diseases should also be excluded.

14. Answer: C

Torticollis

The congenital form is the most common, and can be due to positional or muscular problems, hemivertebrae, unilateral atlanto-axial fusion, Klippel–Feil syndrome and pterygium colli. There are many neurological causes, including Wilson's disease, syringomyelia, cervical tumours, visual disturbance and spinal cord tumours. Trauma and inflammatory disease can also lead to torticollis.

15. Answer: C

16. Answer: B

Polydactyly

Meckel–Gruber syndrome, polysyndactyly and orofaciodigital syndrome are also all associated with polydactyly. Many syndromes are associated with syndactyly, including Apert's, Carpenter's, Cornetia de Lange, Holt–Oram, Laurence–Moon–Biedl, Fanconi's and fetal hydantoin syndromes and trisomies 13, 18 and 21.

17–21. Answers:

17. **C:** The diagnosis of Juvenile chronic arthritis (JCA) can be made in patients under 16 years of age. In addition, the symptoms should have persisted for at least 6 weeks–3 months. There are three types of JCA:

- Pauciarticular-onset JCA – four or fewer joints, which is the most common variety (60–70%).
- Polyarticular-onset JCA – five or more joints affected, which comprises approximately 15–25% of cases.
- Systemic-onset JCA, which includes approximately 20% of patients and is closely associated with temperatures up to 39.5 °C for at least 2 weeks, with or without a typical rash.

The incidence of JCA is approximately 9–25 out of 100 000, with a prevalence of approximately 12–113 per 100 000. The female-to-male ratio is between 2 : 1 and 3 : 1.

A numer of case of pauciarticular-onset JCA may evolve into juvenile spondyloarthropathy or psoriasis. The majority of these patients present between 1 and 3 years of age. This happens more frequently in females, with limping as the initial presentation. It is rarely associated with significant fevers or constitutional symptoms. The knee joints are involved in approximately 50%, but the ankles, elbows and small joints of the hand can also be involved. Between 40% and 75% may have anti-nuclear antibodies (ANAs), and they are frequently associated with a chronic eye disease, namely uveitis, especially if the child is female and under 2 years with positive ANAs. A slit-lamp eye examination is mandatory for all children with JCA. There is also a greater association with sacroiliitis and spondyloarthropathy with enthesopathy. The HLA-B27 gene subtype is associated with these groups of patients, and iritis is common in this group.

Polyarticular-onset JCA occurs in 20% of children with JCA. A group of these are rheumatoid factor IgM-positive, and they can resemble adult-onset arthritis in pattern. The majority are usually female and present between 12 and 16 years of age with symmetrical small-joint involvement, flexor tenosynovitis and nodules commonly being seen. Systemic features are less common in this group. Active disease in adulthood will be more common in these groups. Extra-articular manifestations include lung, cardiac, aortic and vascular disease. In those patients with polyarticular JCA who are seronegative for rheumatoid factor, there is hepatosplenomegaly with fever and symmetrical arthritis. Hip, neck, hand and feet joints are commonly affected, as well as the knees, wrists and ankles. Soft tissue swelling is commonly seen on X-ray, while erosions can be seen in the polyarticular variety. Systemic involvement is seen especially in the pauciarticular and systemic disease subtypes. A blood count can be performed, which will show anaemia of chronic disease, a high ferritin level, thrombocytosis and sometimes thrombocytopenia. The white cell count can be elevated, and mild proteinuria can be identified in 20–40% of cases. The ESR is usually elevated, which does not necessarily correlate with the clinical presentation of the disease. Rheumatoid factors are usually present in 15–20% of thesechildren, in particular those with late-onset polyarticular juvenile chronic arthritis. ANAs are seen in 40–60% of the pauciarticular variety. Technetium bone scans can be used and have proved to be helpful in early diagnosis when X-rays and blood tests are normal.

18. **G:** Systemic-onset JCA is one of the more serious type of JCA, with significant morbidity and mortality. It is associated with fever that rises to 39.5 °C for the first 2 days before the diagnosis is made. Fever occurs late in the afternoon or evening and returns to normal, or below normal, in the morning. The child looks ill and miserable, with a coloured skin rash on the trunk and thighs. The rash may sometimes be itchy. Up to three-quarters of patients will have enlarged lymph nodes, spleen and liver. Pericardial and myocardial involvement may also occur in the form of serositis. Pulmonary disease can occur, with infiltrates, pleurisy and pulmonary fibrosis. Arthritis occurs in approximately three-quarters of cases and usually involves the wrists, knees and ankles, but the temporomandibular joints and hands can also be affected. The condition usually lasts between 2 and 5 years before remitting.

19. **K:** Ankylosing spondylitis is one of a group of diseases – spondyloarthropathies – which also includes arthritis following inflammatory bowel diseases and chronic reactive arthritis following enteric or genitourinary tract infection. They are characterized by inflammation of the joints and involvement of the axial skeleton. Enthesitis is present and characterized by inflammation at the sites of attachment of ligaments, tendons, fascies and capsules. The diagnosis of a spondyloarthropathy is suggested by onset in an older child with oligoarthritis affecting the hips, knees or ankles and accompanied by enthesitis. Radiographic evidence will help in diagnosing ankylosing spondylitis, and shows evidence of sacroiliitis in the form of extensive sclerosis, erosions of joint margins and apparent widening of the joint space. HLA-B27 occurs in 90% of patients with juvenile ankylosing spondylitis (JAS). The ESR can be high. Iridocyclitis occurs in a quarter of patients with JAS. Controlling pain and minimizing inflammation is the treatment target for these patents.

20. **D:** Juvenile dermatomyositis is the most common inflammatory myopathy in children. The gene related to HLA-DQA1*0501 is found in 80% of patients with JDM. It can progress slowly with fatiguability, a low-grade fever and loss of weight, all of which are common. The rash usually appears first over exposed areas, followed by proximal weakness. Periorbital violaceous (heliotropic) erythema occurs across the nasal bridge and around the eyelids. It may involve the upper torso, hands and especially the knuckles. Facial oedema is common. Creatinine kinase will be very high, and aldolase, serum aspartate aminotransferase (AST) and

lactate dehydrogenase (LDH) will be high, but not specific. An MRI scan is also helpful in diagnosis by using T2-weighted images and fat suppression. This will show the active site of the disease, helping muscle biopsy and EMG testing. Corticosteroids, methotrexate and cyclosporine can be used in management. Long-term complications are calcification and calcified nodules with cardiomyopathies.

21. **H:** Behçet's disease is a multisystem disorder with recurrent oral and genital ulceration, relapsing iritis and uveitis, along with cutaneous, arthritic, neurological, vascular and gastrointestinal manifestations. No cause may be found, and it can be associated with HLA-B5 and -B51. Painful ulcers occur in all patients and persist for days and weeks. The condition is uncommon in children, with an overall occurrence of less than 5%. Treatment with corticosteroids, colchicine, chlorambucil, azathioprine and cyclosporine have been tried, and anecdotal results have been reported.

22–26. Answers:

22. D, B, A, G, I, M
23. D, B, A, G, F, I, J, N
24. D, B, I, J, K, L
25. E
26. E, B, A

27–31. Answers:

27. **K:** Developmental dysplasia of the hip (DDH) is one of the neonatal problems that can be postnatal in origin. There are two forms: one is neurologically normal babies and one is babies with underlying neuromuscular disorders. The latter usually occurs in utero. It occurs more in breech position babies or children with lower limb abnormalities, spine abnormalities or neuromuscular problems. A Barlow test is most reliable for examining the newborn's hips. This is a provocative test performed by dislocating an unstable hip while stabilizing the pelvis with one hand, flexing and adducting the opposite hip with the other hand, and applying posterior force. If the hip is dislocatable, this will be felt, and, after releasing the posterior force, the hip will relocate. Twenty percent of cases are familial, and 60% of babies with DDH are firstborns. Only 1 in 800–1000 has true dislocation. Limitation of hip abduction, limping, a shortened leg and increased creases on the thigh all arouse the suspicion of possible DDH. A hip X-ray should be done anteroposteriorly and in a lateral-like frog position. Ultrasound of the hips provides valuable information and should be done within the first 6 weeks of life; if positive, the infant should be referred to the orthopaedic team.

28. **D:** In Legg–Calvé–Perthes disease, there is avascular necrosis of the capital femoral epiphysis. The cause is unknown, and it presents with painless limping and mild to moderate pain in

the anterior thigh. There is an antalgic gait, muscle spasms and mild restriction of movement spinally on abduction and internal rotation of the hips. Radiological changes are varied, but fragmentation and necrosis of the capital femoral epiphysis are the commonest findings on X-ray. It is a local and self-healing condition if containment is applied whereby the femoral head is contained within the acetabulum, which can be done by non-surgical or surgical procedures.

29. **G:** Congenital scoliosis usually occurs in the first trimester and can be a partial or complete (or mixed) failure of vertebral formation. It is associated with genitourinary abnormalities in one-fifth of cases. Spinal dysraphia is associated with congenital scoliosis in many patients (40%). Children are mainly asymptomatic, but signs of scoliosis become more apparent as the child grows and, if associated with spinal cord abnormalities, may present with an inability to walk or delayed walking. At least a quarter of cases may not show curvature and do not require treatment. Treatment should be given early, with regular follow-up by a specialist.

30. **C:** 'Spondylolysis' is the term used to refer to a defect in the pars interarticularis, the posterior plate of bone that connects the superior and inferior articular facets of a vertebral body. It commonly affects L5 and can be congenital or acquired. Back pain, limping and hamstring muscle spasms may be the presenting features in symptomatic patients. Urinary retention is uncommon. On examination, there may be sacral kyphosis and a reduction in lumbar lordosis. X-ray of the lumbar region should include AP, lateral and oblique views of the lumbosacral vertebrae. An MRI is also needed if there are urinary or neurological symptoms.

31. **H:** Toddler fracture usually represents a spiral fracture of the distal third of the tibia. It may result from a simple fall while running or playing. The initial presentation includes pain, refusal to walk and minimal soft tissue swelling with slight warmth over the area of the fracture. The X-ray may be normal, and a bone scan is not needed. If the X-ray is done 2 weeks later, it will show new bone formation. To relieve the pain, analgesia and application of a long leg cast can be used.

ENT and Ophthalmology

BOFs

1. Under 2 years of age, orbital neoplasm is commonly due to:

   A Metastatic neuroblastoma
   B Haemangioma
   C Optic nerve glioma
   D Rhabdomyosarcoma
   E Osteosarcoma

2. The following are signs of papilloedema except:

   A Deeper pink colour disc
   B Blurred margins
   C Fine disc haemorrhages
   D Elevation of disc
   E None of the above

3. Regarding squints in children, the following are true except:

   A Children do not spontaneously 'grow out' of a squint.
   B The concomitant convergent squint is the commonest type.
   C The eye may become amblyopic and develop a squint if it is covered in the treatment of, for example, facial injury.
   D When a child presents with a squint, the other children in the family should not be examined, as squints are not inherited.
   E Refractive errors are a common cause of strabismus, and by far the commonest is hypermetropia.

4. Which of the following statements is not true:

   A Pseudosquint is common in young children and generally disappears by adulthood.
   B In heterophoria, there is normally no deviation of the eyes.
   C Duane's retraction syndrome is considered a type of concomitant squint.
   D Incomitant squint is much less common than concomitant squint.
   E In hypertrophic concomitant squint, the squinting eye deviates upwards.

5. The following are all treatments of squint except:

A Wearing of spectacles
B Occlusion of non-affected eye
C Anticholinesterase drugs
D Botulinus toxin
E None of the above

6. The following are causes of ptosis and are associated with abnormalities of the fingers and toes except:

A Turner's syndrome
B Congenital ptosis
C Marcus Gunn jaw-winking syndrome
D Horner's syndrome
E Neurogenic ptosis

7. The following are known complications of orbital cellulitis except:

A Meningitis
B Paranasal sinusitis
C Optic atrophy
D Exposure keratitis
E Cavernous sinus thrombosis

8. *Chlamydia* causes which of the following forms of conjunctivitis:

A Swimming pool conjunctivitis
B Inclusion blennorrhoea
C Trachoma
D Ophthalmia neonatorum
E All of the above

9. The following diseases will cause a cherry-red spot in the eyes except:

A Fabry's disease
B Tay–Sachs disease
C Wilson's disease
D Gaucher's disease
E Refsum's syndrome

10. A baby was born at 37 weeks of gestation and was noticed to have a cataract in his right eye and bilateral single palmar creases. His liver was palpable 2 cm below the costal margin, but his spleen was not palpable. His mother had a fever and mild facial rash at 10 weeks of pregnancy that was diagnosed as a viral infection. Which one of the following tests will lead to the most likely diagnosis?

A Karyotyping
B TORCH screen
C Urine reducing substances
D Blood sugar monitoring
E Brain CT scan

11. A two-year-old girl is found to have retinoblastoma in her left eye. The following are all false except:

A A slit-lamp examination of the other eye is likely to detect tumour there as well.
B The prognosis nowadays is good, as the tumour is usually detected and treated early.
C The tumour, by growing between the retina and choroids, causes retinal detachment.
D Metastases are common even in the early stages.
E Death is usually caused by extensive spread to the lungs, bones and liver.

12. Which of the following is a first-choice treatment for retinoblastoma?

A Radiotherapy
B Chemotherapy
C A and B
D Enucleation of the involved eye
E B and D

13. The following are all known causes of cataracts except:

A Marfan's syndrome
B Diabetes
C Hypoparathyroidism
D Osteogenesis imperfecta
E Avitaminosis D

14. A 4-year-old boy is seen in A&E with a 3-hour history of an acutely painful left ear. His temperature is 38°C, it is difficult to examine his left ear because of the pain, his throat is congested and the throat examination is not normal. He has a tender, well-localized swelling over the tip of the sternomastoid process. What is the most likely diagnosis?

A Acute otitis media
B Acute mastoiditis
C Furunculosis
D Acute tonsillitis
E Acute cervical lymphadenitis

15. Which of the following characterize secretory otitis media in children?

A Presentation with painful insidious bilateral deafness.
B Most of these children have recurrent otitis media.
C In up to 80%, their hearing will return to normal by 8 weeks of conservative follow-up.
D Its point prevalence is less than 0.1%.
E It has equal sex incidence.

16. The following statements regarding the diagnosis of deafness are all false except:

A Distraction audiometry in the UK is carried out by the health visitor as one of the routine screening tests at 1 year of age.
B Pure tone audiometry cannot be done until the child will tolerate wearing headphones and respond reliably.
C Brainstem evoked response audiometry is not reliable in the first 6 months of life.
D Otoacoustic emissions can distinguish between conductive deafness and sensorineural deafness.
E Impedance audiometry is not useful if the child has secretory otitis media.

17. A 3-year-old child presents with a 1-week history of unilateral blood-stained nasal discharge. The most likely diagnosis is:

A Bacterial rhinitis
B Viral rhinitis
C Allergic rhinitis
D Foreign body in the nose
E Epistaxis

18. Which one of the following statements is true regarding paranasal sinusitis in children?

A Maxillary sinusitis occurs in children from 3 years upwards.
B Ethmoiditis is rare under the age of 8 years.
C Frontal sinusitis is less common than ethmoiditis and presents in children over 10 years of age.
D Maxillary sinusitis usually presents with severe frontal headache and minimal nasal symptoms.
E Frontal sinusitis, but not ethmoiditis, has a risk of spreading to involve the intracranial structures.

19. The following are false regarding choanal atresia except:

A It is not rare, with an incidence over 1 in 1000 liveborn babies.
B Bilateral atresia is commoner than unilateral.
C As the diagnosis is made clinically, a CT scan is usually not necessary before corrective surgery.
D Any baby with bilateral choanal atresia will need urgent endotracheal intubation.
E Less than 50% of cases are associated with the CHARGE syndrome.

20. Adenoidectomy may be indicated in the following conditions except:

A Airway obstruction in a small child
B Severe persistent nasal obstruction
C Quinsy
D Large adenoids found at tonsillectomy
E Secretory otitis media

21. The following are true regarding angiofibroma of the nasopharynx except:

A It is a benign tumour.
B It presents with nasal blockage and epistaxis.
C It can have intracranial extension.
D It presents in teenage males.
E None of the above.

22. The following are indications for tonsillectomy except:

A Marked enlargement of the tonsils
B Airway obstruction
C Suspicion of lymphoma
D Recurrent acute tonsillitis
E Two or more attacks of peritonsillar abscess

23. Which of the following is not a differential diagnosis for acute tonsillitis?

A Infectious mononucleosis
B Viral pharyngitis
C Herpangina
D Moniliasis
E Epiglotitis

24. Regarding acute tonsillitis, the following are true except:

A In a child with peritonsillitis, examination is difficult but will show the affected tonsil to be very red, covered in pus and pushed laterally.
B Quinsy follows peritonsillitis.
C Rheumatic fever is now very rarely seen as a complication of tonsillitis.
D Amoxicillin is not recommended in acute tonsillitis.
E Airway obstruction usually occurs in children aged 2–3 years.

25. Which of the following statements regarding disorders of voice in children are true:

A Dysphonia is difficulty in producing sound and is usually associated with laryngeal disease.
B Vocal nodules occur at the junction between the anterior third and posterior two-thirds of the vocal cords.
C Polyps of the larynx occur following intubation.
D Laryngeal papillomas are associated with maternal genital warts.
E All of the above.

EMQs

26. Match the following craniofacial abnormalities with the appropriate sentence/description:

  (i) Plagiocephaly
 (ii) Trigonocephaly
(iii) Crouzon's anomaly
 (iv) Treacher Collins' syndrome
  (v) Scaphocephaly
 (vi) Oxycephaly

A Asymmetrical suture closure
B Premature closure of the coronal suture
C Premature closure of the sagittal suture
D Premature closure of the midline metopic suture
E Mandibulofacial dysostosis
F Craniofacial dysostosis
G Hypertelorism

27. Match the following types of conjunctivitis with their most common cause (choose one only):

   (i) Ophthalmia neonatorum
  (ii) Acute purulent conjunctivitis
 (iii) Membranous conjunctivitis
  (iv) Exanthematous conjunctivitis
   (v) Phlyctenular conjunctivitis
  (vi) 'Swimming pool' conjunctivitis
 (vii) Pseudomembranous conjunctivitis

A *Chlamydia*
B Gonococcus
C Tuberculosis
D Allergy to bacteria or toxins
E *Corynebacterium diphtheriae*
F Staphylococcus
G Measles
H HIV
I Staphylococcus, pneumococcus and Koch–Weeks bacillus

28. Match the following diseases with their related manifestations:

   (i) Galactosaemia
  (ii) Albinism
 (iii) Cystinosis
  (iv) Homocystinuria
   (v) Wilson's disease
  (vi) Idiopathic hyperlipaemia
 (vii) Niemann–Pick disease

A Squint
B Kayser–Fleischer ring in the cornea
C Arcus juvenilis
D Cherry red spot
E Pendular nystagmus
F Fine crystals in the cornea
G Bilateral dislocation of the lenses
H Anterior uveitis
I Bilateral cataract

29. **Match each of the following congenital causes of deafness with its most frequently associated feature:**

      (i) Waardenburg's syndrome
     (ii) Klippel–Feil syndrome
    (iii) Alport's syndrome
     (iv) Pendred's syndrome
      (v) Refsum's syndrome
     (vi) Usher's syndrome
    (vii) Jervell and Lange–Nielsen syndrome

    A Goitre
    B Contraction of the visual fields
    C Syncopal attacks
    D White forelock
    E Ataxia
    F Limited head movements
    G Glomerulonephritis

Answers for ENT and Ophthalmology

1. Answer: A

Orbital neoplasm

The most common causes of unilateral proptosis are traumatic orbital haemorrhage, meningocele or neoplasm. Under two years of age, orbital neoplasm is commonly metastatic neuroblastoma. Haemangioma, optic nerve glioma and rhabdomyosarcoma are found in children of all ages.

2. Answer: E

Papilloedema

Papilloedema is the disc abnormality about which the ophthalmologist is most often asked to give an opinion. In papilloedema, the optic disc first becomes a deeper pink colour, with its margins blurred. Fine haemorrhages then develop on the disc and in the surrounding retina, and there is elevation of the disc, which can be made out readily using an indirect ophthalmoscope.

3. Answer: D

Strabismus in children

The visual reflexes become established during the first few years of life, and as full recovery of normal vision can only be brought about within a short time of the development of a squint, satisfactory treatment of strabismus depends upon an early diagnosis. The widespread belief that children may spontaneously 'grow out' of a squint is entirely fallacious and still results in many children being referred for treatment only when it is too late. Although surgical cure may still be possible, after a delayed referral, the squinting eye usually remains amblyopic. The earliest possible diagnosis and treatment of a child with a squint is essential.

The most common type of strabismus is of the concomitant convergent nature associated with a hypermetropic refractive error.

The principal causes of squint are sensory and motor. Sensory barriers include any defect in the afferent visual pathway, such as corneal scarring, cataracts and disease of the retina or optic nerve. Any of these will reduce vision, disturb fusion of the two images and, in a child, may provoke a squint. An important cause in this group is the occlusion of one eye by a pad or bandage during treatment of some other condition. If a child's eye is covered in the treatment of, for example, a corneal ulcer or facial injury, the eye may become amblyopic and a squint may develop very quickly.

Refractive errors are a common cause of strabismus, and by far the commonest is hypermetropia, which produces overconvergence resulting in convergent strabismus. Myopia results in underconvergence, leading to a divergent strabismus. Squint is not caused by anxiety, worry, fear or infectious disease, although a latent squint may manifest itself during some intercurrent illness.

Almost 50% of all squinting children have a family history of squint or refractive error. When a child presents with a squint, other children in the family should be examined.

4. Answer: C

Types of squint in children

The appearance of squint is usually caused by marked epicanthal folds that may be bilateral or unilateral, a small or large interpupillary distance, a broad nasal bridge or facial asymmetry. Pseudosquint is a common condition among young children, but it generally disappears with facial development. Epicanthal folds disappear or reduce spontaneously.

Heterophoria (latent squint) is a condition in which there is extraocular muscle imbalance, and although there is normally no deviation of the eyes, a potential deviation is present.

Incomitant (paralytic) squint is much less common. It may be due to paresis of one of the extraocular muscles (paralytic squint). Dysfunction of the 6th nerve is particularly prone to occur, with external (lateral) rectus weakness. Myogenic lesions, which are congenital anomalies, are associated with musculofacial abnormalities. Duane's retraction syndrome is typical of this group, and in this condition, the external rectus muscle becomes fibrosed and may be associated with enophthalmos and ptosis on eye movement.

Concomitant squint is a condition in which the angle of deviation remains unchanged whatever the direction of the gaze. It can be convergent, divergent, hypertrophic (where the squinting eye turns upwards) or hypotrophic (where it turns downwards). The great majority of concomitant squints are horizontal, but occasionally a squint has both a horizontal and a vertical element. A concomitant squint may be intermittent, being present only on fixation for certain distances or in a certain direction of gaze, but it is generally manifest at all times.

5. Answer: E

Treatment of squint

In the management of squinting in children, occlusion of one eye may produce a rapid improvement in vision. The wearing of spectacles, together with occlusion and orthoptic treatment, may alone be sufficient to correct a squint and restore binocular vision. If this is the case then no further treatment may be necessary. Follow-up is required, as there may be a relapse.

Surgical treatment may be necessary in some cases. Anticholinesterase drugs, such as pilocarpine drops and diisopropylfluorophosphate (DFP), can be used to cause a decrease in accommodation with a corresponding reduction in convergence. These are good for an accommodative type of convergent squint where the initial angle is small and the squint greatest for near vision.

The most recent method of treatment uses an injection of botulinum toxin, which has been used to induce partial and temporary paralysis of an extra-ocular nerve.

6. Answer: B

Ptosis

Ptosis is the most common developmental abnormality of the eyelids, but is not always congenital. It is often an isolated finding and can be associated with other conditions or ocular abnormalities (e.g. epicanthal folds and squint), with remote congenital defects, including abnormalities of the fingers and toes, or as part of Turner's syndrome. Congenital ptosis is usually bilateral and often hereditary.

If there is interference with vision, a surgical approach to correct it will be appropriate. Sympathetic ptosis (Horner's syndrome) results only in slight drooping of the eyelid, and surgery is not usually necessary.

The third nerve can be the cause and the condition can be congenital, when there is often an associated paresis of the superior rectus muscle. The pupil may be fixed and dilated. Mechanical ptosis results from drooping of an eyelid that has been thickened by traumatic or inflammatory scarring.

7. Answer: B

Orbital cellulitis

This is usually pyogenic and in many cases is due to spread of infection from the paranasal sinus (the ethmoid sinus and, in older children, from the ethmoid, frontal or maxillary sinuses). Orbital cellulitis can cause septicaemia with a high temperature, and the child will look toxic. Complications include meningitis, cavernous sinus thrombosis and papilloedema, leading to optic atrophy and exposure keratitis. It usually responds very well to intravenous antibiotics (ceftriaxone or co-amoxiclav) for 5 days.

8. Answer: F

9. Answer: B

Tay–Sachs disease

In Tay–Sachs disease, on ophthalmoscopy there is a cherry-red spot with a grey–white halo of lipid-laden cells that can be seen in the macular region. There is no visceromegaly, but there is usually progressive enlargement of the head from the stored lipids in the brain.

Gaucher's disease

This gives a diffuse white appearance in the fundus, but no cherry-red spot.

Fabry's disease

There are abnormal eye findings that include angioid streaks in the retina and characteristic whorl-like corneal opacities, which may be seen by slit-lamp examination in most hemizygotes and in up to 70% of heterozygotes.

10. Answer: B

Cataracts in newborn babies

Cataracts are found in babies whose mothers contracted the rubella virus infection in the first trimester of pregnancy. They are usually bilateral, and the extent of opacity in both eyes is usually unequal. The entire lens may be opaque, or more commonly there is a dense central opacity with a clearer peripheral area. Live rubella virus has been cultured from lens material removed from such eyes many months after birth. Rubella cataracts respond remarkably well to surgery, although if there is rubella retinopathy, this treatment may not be successful.

Galactosaemia can also cause cataracts, and any baby with a cataract should be screened for this. It is bilateral, appears between the 4th and 8th weeks of life in untreated cases, and increases rapidly until the lens is completely opaque by the 10th week. Where complete lens opacity develops, it is irreversible, but the results of surgery are good.

Diabetic cataracts occur in poorly controlled diabetes, but are very rare. Down's syndrome is commonly associated with cataracts in babies (about 75% of such children have lens opacities). The opacities are generally small and discrete and do not interfere with vision. Regular checks and early treatment will improve vision.

11. Answer: C

Retinoblastoma

Retinoblastoma develops before the 3rd year of life and is rarely congenital. Retinoblastoma is usually hereditary and familial as well as multifocal. Only a quarter are bilateral. It usually starts as a small white area in the fundus or on the retina. It may grow between the retina and choroid and cause secondary retinal detachment, or it may grow inward into the vitreous. Seedlings are common and can spread to other parts of the eye. If untreated, it will cause glaucoma with pain and loss of vision. It can fill the orbit rapidly and spread to the optic nerve, then to the brain and can cause death. It can regress spontaneously in some cases.

12. Answer: D

Treatment of retinoblastoma

Enucleation of the involved eye with the removal of as much of the optic nerve as possible is the treatment of choice, followed by radiotherapy if the optic nerve is affected. Radiation alone can be used if the tumour is discovered early. Children will survive, having a normal life, and regular check-ups for the other eyes every 2 months until the child reaches 10 years of age are ideal and very important. If the other eye is affected, radiotherapy should be applied, as the tumour is radiosensitive. Some children with retinoblastoma treated with radiation develop sarcoma in or around the orbit in early adult life, and all children with retinoblastoma treated by radiation should be kept under supervision indefinitely. Because of the genetic associations, families with this tumour require genetic counselling.

13. Answer: A

Hypoparathyroid cataracts are bilateral, subcapsular opacities developing as lamellae in the lens, each of which corresponds to an attack of tetany. If the condition is untreated, the lens opacity progresses towards maturity, but with successful treatment there is no further opacification, although the isolated lamellae of opacity remain unchanged.

Avitaminosis D in early infancy produces bilateral lamellar cataracts. A clear lens develops outside the areas of opacification when the deficiency is corrected. Avitaminosis D in a mother produces corresponding lamellar cataracts in the fetus that appear as congenital cataracts.

14. Answer: C

Otitis externa

This is not common in children. It can be treated by aural toilet and topical antibiotics with or without steroids. The skin of the meatus is often swollen and extremely tender. Furunculosis can also occur in the external meatus.

Acute otitis media

This is commonly associated with URTI and other infections. It can present as an acutely painful ear and is usually bilateral, and the child will be febrile and may develop febrile convulsions. If the eardrum is inspected, it will appear either acutely inflamed or bulging with obvious pus behind it; the pain is due to build-up of mucopurulent secretions in the middle ear. Analgesia and antibiotics, in some cases, will help to clear it up. If it is recurrent, the child should be referred to an ENT specialist.

Acute mastoiditis

This will present with an acutely tender swelling in the postauricular region, with the area of maximum tenderness being over the surface marking of the mastoid, which is at the level of the top of the tragus. The ear may or may not be discharging. The child will usually be in considerable pain and will be febrile.

15. Answer: A

Secretory otitis media

This is a very common condition, affecting children between age 4 and 6 years and is more common in boys. It usually presents with painless insidious bilateral conductive deafness. The problem may not be identified until routine audiometric testing is performed at school. The fluid collects due to blockage of the eustachian tube. If children are left for up to 8 weeks, 20% of them will drain their fluid, and their hearing will return to normal. If clearance of the fluid does not occur within 2 months, the only available treatment is surgical. Surgery consists of myringotomy (drainage of the fluid) with adenoidectomy, with grommet tube insertion, or with both.

16. Answer: B

Distraction audiometry can be performed at 7–8 months of age when the child can hold his head in the middle. It is still a reliable, efficient method of testing and requires minimal equipment. Pure-tone audiometry is the main method of testing, but cannot be done until the child will tolerate wearing headphones and can be relied upon to respond accurately to pure-tone sounds, usually at around 5–6 years of age.

Brainstem evoked response audiometry is the most reliable form of objective audiometry and can be performed at any age. Its disadvantages are that it takes a considerable time, it is not frequency-specific and the child will have to be lying quietly or sedated for it to be performed satisfactorily.

Otoacoustic emissions are a quick, efficient and very simple form of objective audiometry that is increasingly being suggested as the most useful test for screening children. Its disadvantages are that it does not distinguish between conductive deafness and sensorineural deafness and that any children who fail the otoacoustic emission test usually then have to progress to brainstem evoked response audiometry.

Impedance audiometry or tympanometry is a simple test that measures the compliance of the eardrum and the pressure of the air in the middle ear. It is ideally suited for identifying secretory otitis media patients and is useful in screening outpatients who have failed their routine school audiometric testing.

17. Answer: D

Blood-stained nasal discharge

A foreign body is one of the causes of unilateral, foul, smelly and blood-stained nasal discharge. This occurs most often in children between the ages of 2 and 4 years.

Epistaxis is very common at any age, and it can be spontaneous or as a result of any trauma. Exclusion of blood disorders is important, and seeking specialist opinion is very important if it becomes frequent. Viral rhinitis and bacterial rhinitis can also present with nasal discharge.

Allergic rhinitis usually occurs in children over 5 years old. It presents as sneezing and is associated with clear rhinorrhoea, nasal blockage, often conjunctivitis and sore throat. Confirmation of the allergic basis can be made by carrying out skin testing or sending RAST IgE for possible allergen.

18. Answer: C

The paranasal sinuses

The paranasal sinuses (maxillary, ethmoid, frontal and sphenoid) are all derived from the nasal cavity and are lined with respiratory epithelium. The maxillary sinuses are small at birth and do not attain a significant size until 4 or 5 years of age. The ethmoid sinuses are well developed at birth, but the frontal sinuses do not develop until 9 or 10 years old. The sphenoid sinuses rarely cause symptoms in childhood.

Maxillary sinusitis is rare under the age of 6 years, and usually follows influenza or parainfluenza. Ethmoiditis is a potentially serious condition, which occurs in children from 3 years upwards. Treatment should be with antibiotics, and it is important that a CT scan be done to confirm the diagnosis.

Frontal sinusitis is less common than ethmoiditis and presents in children over 10 years of age. Like ethmoiditis, it is potentially serious, with a risk of spreading to involve the orbit or intracranial structures.

19. Answer: E

Choanal atresia

More than half of these cases are associated with CHARGE syndrome. It can be bilateral, and is a neonatal emergency. It can be suspected in a baby who breathes normally and is not a mouth breather but who collapses everytime whether fed or not. Passing a nasal tube will be difficult. Establishing an airway is important with a CT scan to determine to what extent and referral to specialist.

20. Answer: C

21. Answer: E

Angiofibroma

Angiofibroma is a benign tumour at the back of the nose and nasopharynx. It can affect teenagers and is more common in males. It is usually noted with nasal blockage and epistaxis. If extended to the back, it may compress the cranial nerves. MRI and CT scans will help in diagnosis. After the diagnosis is confirmed, treatment is by surgery initially, radiotherapy being reserved for intracranial extension.

22. Answer: A

Indications for tonsillectomy

Enlargement of the tonsils on their own is not an indication for their removal, but airway obstruction is an absolute indication in small children with persistent noisy breathing and suspected or proven sleep apnoea. The adenoids will also be removed. Suspicion of other pathology (e.g. lymphoma) is also an absolute indication. Recurrent acute tonsillitis is another. If a child is having six or seven attacks of definite tonsillitis in 1 year or five attacks per year for 2 years, this is an indication for adenotonsillectomy. Two or more attacks of peritonsillar abscess is another indication.

23. Answer: D

Infectious mononucleosis occurs in older children and is often accompanied by marked lymphadenopathy in the neck and other areas. The child is miserable, with throat discomfort due to generalized congestion of the throat and swelling of the tonsils. Serological confirmation can resolve doubt, and treatment is supportive with analgesia and fluids. In viral pharyngitis, the child is less ill and has other symptoms, e.g. blocked nose or red congested throat and no pus on the tonsils. Herpangina is a self-limiting condition due to infection by the coxsackievirus, and has papular, vesicular and ulcerative lesions on the anterior pillars, palate and tonsils. Moniliasis is characterized by white patches that are present on the tongue, tonsils and pharynx.

24. Answer: A

In mild tonsillitis, analgesia and adequate fluid intake are all that is required, but in more severe cases penicillin V for 7–10 days is usually successful. Erythromycin may be used where there is a penicillin sensitivity. Amoxicillin or co-amoxiclav are less suitable and are not suitable if given to a child with mononucleosis.

Peritonsillar abscess (quinsy) is less common in children. It can occur during or just after an acute attack of tonsillitis, and presents with increasing pain and swelling, usually on one side of the throat, with marked dysphagia and often otalgia. The child will have difficulty in opening his/her mouth. Examination is difficult, but will show the affected tonsil to be very red, covered in pus and pushed medially. In addition, there will be gross swelling and redness of the palate and marked cervical lymphadenopathy on the ipsilateral side. If untreated, the abscess can spread to give rise to a parapharyngeal abscess, with the risk of spread to the base of the skull or even into the superior mediastinum. Treatment is drainage under general anaesthetic, which can be a hazardous procedure. If it is not certain that pus is present, intravenous penicillin or erythromycin is given with fluids and analgesics.

Airway obstruction usually occurs in children aged 2–3 years as a result of chronic hypertrophy of the adenoids and tonsils. The child breathes noisily at night (and occasionally stops breathing for short periods) and often during the day. If untreated, this relatively common complication of tonsillitis can lead to chronic hypoxia, pulmonary hypertension and, in severe cases, core pulmonale. Where there is any suggestion of airway obstruction, a sleep study with monitoring of oxygen saturation is needed. If there are episodes of desaturation indicative of sleep apnoea, adenotonsillectomy is indicated. Such children should be admitted to the high-dependency unit on the night of surgery, and their breathing pattern should be monitored, as their respiratory drive may be depressed.

Rheumatic fever is now very rarely seen as a complication of tonsillitis.

25. Answer: E

Dysphonia, or difficulty in producing sound, is usually associated with laryngeal disease (hoarseness). It may follow a URTI, and the voice will recover. Persistent hoarseness should be investigated, and this can only be done by visualization of the larynx with a fibre-optic endoscope passed along the nose into the nasopharynx. Where this is not possible, direct laryngoscopy is indicated to define the pathology. The causes of hoarseness in children are vocal nodules, polyps of the larynx and laryngeal papilloma (this is a rare cause of hoarseness associated with maternal genital warts (papillomavirus)) and unilateral vocal cord paralysis (which can follow surgical or non-surgical trauma to the neck).

26. Answers:

(i) A
(ii) D
(iii) F
(iv) E
(v) C
(vi) B

Craniostenosis

Oxycephaly (tower skull) is caused by premature closure of the coronal suture, resulting in a high skull with a steep forehead.

Scaphocephaly (boat-shaped skull) is caused by premature closure of the sagittal suture.

Plagiocephaly is due to asymmetrical suture closure.

Trigonocephaly is caused by premature closure of the midline metopic suture of the frontal bone, resulting in a triangular-shaped skull.

The craniostenoses are frequently of a minor degree and cause only a cosmetic defect, but where they are more advanced, they may result in raised intracranial pressure, often indicated by papilloedema. They will then need prompt surgical decompression of the skull or optic foramina before optic atrophy develops.

Cranial dysostosis

Craniofacial dysostosis (Crouzon's anomaly) is a hereditary association of oxycephaly, shallow orbits and aplasia of the maxilla, with nasal and palatal defects. Shallow orbits may result in proptosis with corneal exposure, and this may necessitate orbital decompression.

Mandibulofacial dysostosis (Treacher Collins' syndrome or Franceschetti's syndrome) includes malformations of the eyelids and ears, with hypoplasia of the bones of the face and sometimes colobomas of the eyelids and iris or fundus.

Hypertelorism is a hereditary developmental anomaly in which the orbits are widely separated and other anomalies generally coexist together with mental retardation.

27. Answers:

   (i) B
  (ii) F
 (iii) E
 (iv) G
  (v) D
 (vi) A
(vii) I

Conjunctivitis

Conjunctivitis is inflammation of the mucous membrane lining the eyelids and the globe of the eye; it is generally infective, but may be due to chemicals, trauma, a foreign body or allergic in origin. Epidemics of conjunctivitis are common among schoolchildren.

In acute purulent conjunctivitis, there is a copious discharge of mucus and pus, and there is systemic toxicity. The causative organism is frequently a staphylococcus, but other pyogenic organisms may be responsible.

Ophthalmia neonatorum is an acute purulent conjunctivitis of the newborn, which may be due to gonococci. Severe untreated cases may cause blindness. *Chlamydia trachomatis* is another common cause.

Membranous conjunctivitis is rare nowadays and is generally due to *Corynebacterium diphtheriae*. Pseudomembranous conjunctivitis is also rare, although it occurs more frequently than diphtheritic conjunctivitis, and is caused by a number of organisms, including staphylococci, pneumococci and Koch–Weeks bacillus.

Exanthematous conjunctivitis occurs particularly in measles, vaccinia and varicella.

Phlyctenular conjunctivitis is a localized inflammation on one part of the conjunctiva or occasionally the cornea, where a small nodule develops and eventually ulcerates. The cause is probably a local allergy to bacteria or toxins.

Viral conjunctivitis is a large group due to many different organisms. A viral conjunctivitis in which the specific diagnosis can be made. A blennorrhoea is caused by *Chlamydia*, which is pathogenic for the conjunctiva, cervix uteri and male urethra. This causes an apparently simple conjunctivitis in young children or 'swimming pool' conjunctivitis in older children.

Trachoma, caused by *Chlamydia*, is still the greatest cause of preventable blindness in the world and has been identified since the earliest times in warm climates. Treatment can appear to be almost impossible because of appalling conditions of hygiene throughout a whole population, and often the treatment of large groups of people is necessary (e.g. the topical administration of tetracycline twice daily to the population), and at the same time the general hygiene of the community should be improved and insects eliminated.

28. Answers:

(i) I
(ii) E
(iii) F
(iv) G
(v) B
(vi) C
(vii) D

29. Answers:

(i) D
(ii) F
(iii) G
(iv) A
(v) E
(vi) B
(vii) C

There are large numbers of syndromes in which deafness is a recognized factor.

Waardenburg's syndrome is an autosomal dominant condition with variable expression and consists of some or all of the following characteristics: unilateral or bilateral perceptive deafness (20% of cases), hypertrichosis of the eyebrows, which meet in the midline, heterochromia of the irises, or a white forelock.

In Klippel–Feil syndrome, a short neck limits head movements, the hairline is low at the back, there may be paralysis of the external rectus muscle in one or both eyes, and there is perceptive hearing loss that may be severe.

Alport's syndrome is X-linked dominant and affects boys more severely than girls. There is severe progressive glomerulonephritis and a progressive sensorineural loss that does not show itself until the boy is about 10 years old.

Pendred's syndrome is autosomal recessive and causes simple goitre at about the age of 4–5 years. The associated deafness is often severe.

Refsum's syndrome consists of ichthyosis, ataxia, retinitis pigmentosa, night blindness, mental retardation and a sensorineural deafness.

Usher's syndrome is autosomal recessive. There is retinitis pigmentosa with contraction of the visual fields and a severe sensorineural loss that may be progressive.

Jervell and Lange-Nielsen syndrome is autosomal recessive with cardiac arrhythmia and profound sensorineural deafness. These children may present with syncopal attacks, which if untreated, can be fatal.

Dermatology

BOFs

1. The following disorders are associated with vesiculobullous lesions:

    A Erythema toxicum
    B Candidiosis
    C Molluscum contagiosum
    D Scabies
    E Erythema multiforme

2. Which of the followings drugs may cause Stevens–Johnson syndrome?

    A Cephalosporins
    B Isoniazid
    C Tetracycline
    D Penicillin
    E Erythromycin

3. The following are true about epidermolysis bullosa except:

    A Epidermolysis bullosa simplex is inherited as an autosomal dominant disorder.
    B Junctional epidermolysis bullosa is lethal.
    C Squamous cell carcinoma is associated with epidermolysis bullosa simplex.
    D Marked deformity of the hands and feet is associated with dystrophic epidermolysis bullosa.
    E Dysplastic teeth, pyloric stricture and loss of nails are features of junctional epidermolysis bullosa.

4. The following are true about atopic dermatitis except:

    A It is inherited as an autosomal dominant disorder.
    B It is characterized by weeping, oozing and itching in the acute phase.
    C Dry and scaly skin can be found.
    D There is a high level of IgE.
    E There is a tendency to remission at age 3–5 years.

5. The following are common benign skin lesions in neonates except:

    A Cutis maramata
    B Naevus simplex (salmon patch)
    C Erythema toxicum
    D Transient pustular melanosis
    E Aplastic cutis congenita

6. Which of the following is associated with skin nodules:

    A Neurofibroma
    B Dermoid
    C Exostosis
    D Haemangioma
    E Xanthoma

7. The differential diagnosis of nappy rash includes all of the following except:

    A Congenital syphilis
    B Scabies
    C Wiskott–Aldrich syndrome
    D Impetigo
    E Psoriasis

8. The following skin lesions are matched correctly with their causative organism except:

    A Warts: human papillomavirus
    B Molluscum contagiosum: poxvirus
    C Genital warts: human papillomavirus type 11
    D Genital herpes simplex: herpes simplex virus type II
    E Lyme disease: *Borrelia burgdorferi*

9. Which of the following drugs is matched correctly with the treated condition:

    A Benzyl benzoate: head lice
    B Benzyl peroxide: acne
    C Dithranol: psoriasis
    D Podophyllin: genital warts
    E Griseofulvin: tinea capitis

10. The following are the most common causes of diffuse alopecia except:

    A Progeria
    B Ectodermal dysplasia
    C Aplasia cutis
    D Hypothyroidism
    E Cockayne's disease

11. The following skin lesions are all associated with SLE except:

   A Butterfly rash
   B Livedo reticularis
   C Photosensitivity
   D Calcinosis
   E Urticaria

12. Cutaneous manifestations associated with diabetes mellitus include:

   A Xanthomas
   B Necrobiosis lipoidica
   C Disseminated granuloma annulare
   D Generalized pruritis
   E Raynaud's phenomenon

EMQs

13–17. From the description of the followings conditions, select the most
   appropriate diagnoses from the list below:

   13. An 8-year-old child has a hyperpigmented patch on his left
   upper thigh that is oval in shape and about 5×6 cm. There
   are four similar to this on his back, buttocks and shoulder.
   He also has a smaller one in his axilla. Eye examinations are
   reported as abnormal, and he is referred to a specialist.

   14. A 3-month-old is seen in Casualty, as his mother is anxious
   that a dark blue lesion has appeared on his back and is more
   obvious than before. She was told by her health visitor to
   take the child to hospital, and the health visitor wrote a letter
   saying to rule out NAI. The lesion over the right buttock is
   bluish-black and macular. Both of his parents are from India.

   15. A 12-month-old infant has developed a large, rubbery
   nodule over his left scapula over the last 4 months. The
   overlying skin is normal in colour, and ultrasound shows
   large vascular elements.

   16. A 3-year-old has been seen several times with a diagnosis of
   eczema, but his condition has never been under control. The
   lesions are red plaques covered with silvery scales. The child
   had a throat infection when this started 10 months ago. It is
   mainly affecting the extensor part of his body.

   17. A 12-year-old boy presents with annular lesions with
   central clearing and an itchy, palpable, erythematous,
   advancing edge with some vesicular and pustular lesions
   nearer the margins. His parents own two cats and a dog.

Options
A   Tuberous sclerosis
B   Mongolian blue spots
C   Eczema
D   Tinea corporis
E   Neurofibromatosis
F   Porphyria
G   Papular urticaria
H   Acne
I   Psoriasis
J   Pityriasis rubra pilaris
K   Vascular naevi
L   Cavernous haemangioma
M   Herpes zoster
N   Impetigo

18–20. The following conditions are associated with skin lesions in neonates. Select the most appropriate test to reach the diagnosis from the list below:

18. A 5-day-old baby was brought to a family doctor, who made a diagnosis of staphylococcal infection and sent him to hospital for intravenous antibiotics. The lesions are blotchy macular erythemas with tiny yellow or white papules.

19. A 2-week-old baby was seen in causality with pustular lesions on the scalp, hands and feet. A sample from one of these was taken to the laboratory for microscopy and culture. Microscopic examination revealed a large number of eosinophils and neutrophils, no organisms, and a negative culture after 5 days. The lesions disappeared, and the parents returned within a week to the hospital and were reassured again.

20. A 3-day-old baby has superficial vesicular and pustular eruptions on his face and trunk. They are weepy, but the baby is still feeding well. The skin has started to show some desquamation on the neck.

Options
A   Skin swab
B   Blood culture
C   Immunoglobulin level
D   C-reactive protein
E   Full blood count
F   IgE level
G   Nothing
H   C3 and C4 complement
I   PCR for HIV
J   Lumbar puncture
K   Rubella IgM
L   PCR for HSV
M   Abdominal US

Answers for Dermatology

1. Answer: C

Vesiculobullous lesions

There are many conditions associated with vesiculobullous lesions, including acrodermatitis enteropathica, insect bites, pemphigus vulgaris, *Pseudomonas* skin infections, syphilis, viral blisters, mastocytosis, eczema herpaticum, dystrophic eczema, bullous impetigo, incontinentia pigmenti, scalded skin syndrome and toxic epidermal necrolysis.

2. Answer: E

Drugs that can cause Stevens–Johnson syndrome

Other drugs include phenytoin, lamotrigine, carbamazepine, valproic acid, sulfonamides and quinolones. Viruses such as herpes, EBV, hepatitis, herpes simplex, and enteroviruses, as well as mycoplasmas and group B streptococci can also cause this syndrome.

3. Answer: C

Epidermolysis bullosa

Junctional epidermolysis bullosa is lethal; it is an autosomal recessive type with localized or progressive scarring, and can affect the mucosa. The simplex type involves hands and feet, with less mucosal involvement and no scarring. The dystrophic type is inherited as an autosomal recessive disorder, is usually associated with aggressive squamous cell carcinoma of the skin, tongue and oesophagus, and can cause many strictures when mucosal surfaces are involved. The dominant dystrophic type is usually associated with hyperkeratotic lesions and squamous cell carcinoma.

4. Answer: A

Atopic dermatitis

This is an inflammatory skin disorder characterized by erythema, intense pruritis, exudation, crusting and scaling. There is usually a family history of asthma, hayfever or allergic rhinitis. More than 80% of cases have serum IgE increased by 5–10-fold. Eosinophilia will support the diagnosis. Flexure lichenification with facial and extensor involvement is typical. Environmental control and application of emulsified creams with or without hydrocortisone are methods for controlling it, and many cases will clear by the age of 3–5 years.

5. Answer: E

Benign skin lesions in neonates

Eosinophilic pustular folliculitis, milia, Mongolian spots, sucking blisters, harlequin colour and infantile acropustulosis are normal, benign and transient skin lesions during the neonatal period.

6. Answer: E

Skin nodules

Xanthoma is a yellowish papule or nodule that contains lipid-filled histocytic cells. These lesions reflect hyperlipidaemia. It is rare in infancy and childhood. It can be secondary to diabetes mellitus, myxoedema, nephritic syndrome and biliary tract obstruction. Other conditions associated with nodules include mastocytoma, juvenile xanthogranuloma, neurofibroma, angiolipoma, leiomyoma, pilomatrixoma, keloids, rheumatoid nodules, histocytosis X and pyogenic granuloma.

7. Answer: D

Nappy rash

Other causes include atopic eczema, Letterer–Siwe disease, acquired zinc deficiency, Kawasaki's disease and acrodermatitis enteropathica. Nappy rash is a form of acute irritant contact dermatitis due to occlusive contact of urine and faeces with skin. Ammonia from breakdown of bacteria will cause this. Nappy rash is also caused by skin wetness, friction, irritant faeces and urine and bacteria. The skin is moist and angry and the condition can sometimes be papuloerosive with ulceration called Jacquet's ulcers. Skin fold not affected. Candidiasis is common, with bright red scaly skin surrounding discrete satellite lesions and with involvement of skin folds.

8. Answer: D

Genital herpes simplex is caused by HSV type I, is usually sexually transmitted, and may affect the penis, vulva or cervix. Topical aciclovir is the treatment of choice, and children at risk should receive it intravenously.

9. Answer: A

Benzyl benzoate is used to treat scabies. Head lice is treated with a frequent fine tooth comb and malathion.

10. Answer: C

Alopecia

Aplasia cutis can cause patch alopecia with scarring, as can burns, trauma, X-rays, morphoea, lichen planus, discoid lupus, incontinentia pigmenti and epidermal naevi. The causes of batch alopecia without scarring include alopecia arreata, trauma, tinea capitis, psoriasis and lichen simplex.

11. Answer: D

Skin lesions associated with SLE

Other lessions include Raynaud's phenomenon, petechiae, purpura and chilblain-like lesions.

12. Answer: E

Skin lesions associated with diabetes mellitus

Others include candidiasis and staphylococcal infection as recurrent boils.

13. Answer: E

As well as in neurofibromatosis, café-au-lait spots can also be found in tuberous sclerosis and Albright–McCune syndrome. NF1 can be diagnosed with six café-au-lait patches of >15 mm post-pubertal and >6 mm pre-pubertal plus three of the following: family history, axillary freckling, Lisch nodules, bone abnormalities or optic glioma.

14. Answer: B

Mongolian blue spots occur in people originally from the Far East or of oriental origin. It is benign, fades slowly over the first year of life, and can be mistaken as a bruise by people who have not seen it before.

15. Answer: L

Cavernous haemangiomas have a rubbery feeling and can be associated with skin changes, such as strawberry naevi. They usually disappear before school age, and with cosmetic surgery have a very good outcome.

16. Answer: I

Psoriasis is a chronic, relapsing, inflammatory skin condition, which is usually familial and affects adults more than children. The onset may be related to a streptococcal throat infection (guttate psoriasis), otitis media, vaccination, insect bites or trauma. It is more common in girls, and early onset is associated with a poor prognosis. Ultraviolet, tar, salicylic acid, dithranol, topical steroids, methotrexate, vitamin A analogues and photochemotherapy can all be used in the treatment of all forms of psoriasis.

17. Answer: D

Tinea corporis is a dermatophyte infection by filamentous fungi that are usually found in the outer layer of the skin. It usually affects skin, but any part of the body can be affected with different types of these fungi. Microscopic examination is important, and a sensitivity test is required. Imidazoles can be used for 4 weeks, and itraconazole is effective, as is Whitfield's ointment (compound benzoic acid ointment).

18. Answer: G

Erythema toxicum is a generalized blotchy macular erythema with tiny yellow or white papules. It is seen from the first week of life up to 6 weeks of age. There is accumulation of eosinophils and the condition usually disappears slowly.

19. Answer: G

Acropustulosis of infancy has an unknown aetiology, with pustules on the scalp, feet and hands. It appears at birth or during the first few weeks of life. They are sterile with a well baby and heal within 5–6 days.

20. Answers: A, B, D, E

Impetigo neonatorum appears in the 2nd or 3rd day of life. It is usually due to staphylococcal infection and may be followed by extensive desquamation. It is important to provide antibiotics, adequate hydration and skin care.